the

DANGEROUS
MIND *of a*
DYING MAN

JASON KOM-TONG

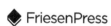 FriesenPress

One Printers Way
Altona, MB R0G 0B0
Canada

www.friesenpress.com

Copyright © 2021 by Jason Kom-Tong
First Edition — 2021

ISBN
978-1-5255-6415-4 (Hardcover)
978-1-5255-6416-1 (Paperback)
978-1-5255-6417-8 (eBook)

1. BIOGRAPHY & AUTOBIOGRAPHY, MEDICAL

Distributed to the trade by The Ingram Book Company

Table of Contents

PROLOGUE

Before I share my life with you, I need to forewarn you that my story is not about how I beat cancer, because even though I am now considered cancer-free/stable, I did not *beat* cancer. The truth is that cancer beat the crap out of me. And it won. Even to this day, just to keep it at bay, I must do monthly treatments. And there is no end in sight.

That's the reason I started writing my story. It was supposed to be only for my kids' eyes. That way, even if I died, they would know the lessons I learned and my advice for situations that would come up in their own lives. My story has no filter and documents all the real-life struggles I went through before, during, and after what was to be my death sentence.

Cancer changed me not only physically but mentally. Indeed, I almost turned into someone who was everything I was not. Survival is a funny thing—you never know how much of a fight you have in you until you're faced with the challenge of making life-or-death decisions that affect your loved ones. For example, *this* decision to put myself and my whole life out there for the world to see. My decision to publish this book and show everyone my shames, mistakes, devious behaviors, deepest fears, and most wrenching regrets was not one I took lightly. To be honest, having everyone know my story scares the shit out of me. I could walk through a grocery store and total strangers may know everything about me, both the good and the terrible. But upon weighing my considerations, I felt my story needed to be made public, just so people could get a better understanding of real-life fears they may need to face themselves one day. When you are pushed into a corner, you sometimes have no option and must do what you have to do to survive. And when an opportunity presents itself, you need to grab on to it and never look back.

Regardless of what happens to me after my story goes out, the most important thing is that it'll be on paper for my kids to read, a record of what I learned in my life to direct them along the right paths. They need to know all about their dad, both the good and the bad, to understand where I am today and why I have a second chance at life. Though I would have made some decisions differently had I had another swing at them, I need my kids to know the man I was and how we got to where we are. And to know that I do everything for them.

Their survival is more important to me than my own, so putting my future on the line of either living my last days behind bars in a maximum-security prison or living them out selfishly with my loved ones surrounding me and doing all I can for them, right down to my dying breaths, was a no-brainer. I blindly threw my future to the wolves and prayed I could get away with it long enough to die before being caught. But as time passed while I was planning all this, it became apparent that my death wasn't as imminent as I'd thought. As my health improved, so did my plans. And this led me to where I am today, which is the launch of my company.

Please be warned that a lot of my story will be hard for many people to read, and it will be difficult to grasp how much heartache it contains and what's entailed in truly putting what's left of your life on the line. But in the final conclusion, you will see how it was 100% worth it in my mind. My survival is through my children, not through me anymore. So, once I realized that the entire rulebook of my life had changed, I did what I felt was best for my family.

Kids, please be wary of what you are about to hear about me. At least you know the true person your dad was and the upbringing that drove him to the decisions he's made and still makes.

About me:

I won't lie and say I had the perfect life before the cancer, because that's just not true. I made some major mistakes along the way. But you need to know what I did and didn't do to understand the morals I have instilled in me and the way I want my children to live their lives. Many of the lessons I didn't fully appreciate until after I was terminal, when I spent months on end in a hospital bed with nothing to do but think back on my life. It was then I realized what really mattered to me and what I would have done differently. As time passed and my life expectancy was increased, I realized I could use this story to help repair many of my regrets. These stories are my life experiences and what I learned from them, and I share them through my eyes. When cancer took my tongue, I figured the best way to pass them on was to write a book about everything and how it changed me, both physically and mentally.

Initially, telling my story for others to hear (besides my kids) never crossed my mind. But after many people approached me for advice on how I had been able to beat cancer, I figured it would be best to write it all down. That way, others could understand the struggles and emotions one goes through in such scenarios and why I did what I did to become who I am today.

Honestly, what surprised me the most when people approached me was that most of them didn't actually want to hear my *real* story. They wanted to hear how life is now rainbows and roses. They didn't want to know about the real-life struggles and mental state a person in my situation suffers. They only wanted to hear about my treatments, recovery, and—of course—my secret to being the only one in my medical trial to survive Stage 4 squamous cell carcinoma of the tongue. They wanted me to sing about how life is so perfect for me now that I've survived!

The fact is that, yes, I really *am* grateful to be alive today. But my life is far from roses and butterflies. In fact, I struggle every day, and if it wasn't for my amazing wife and kids, I would probably not be or want to be alive today. So if you are looking for a nice story about rainbows and fluffy clouds, this is not the one for you. This is the one that's about how someone following what he believed to be the right life path met cancer there and was led down a dark offshoot. The one about the battle I had to go through and the things I was willing to do to get out of the darkness. In the end, I was put on a different path, which turned out to be the one I was supposed to be following my whole life, the one that would teach me to know real happiness.

My story may be hard to follow at times, but if you can, you will understand my life and what I learned along the way.

Writing this was very difficult for me because, as we all know, life doesn't flow nicely past, chapter by chapter. It's complicated and full of emotions. Multiple things overlap and most of us live lives filled with a spiderweb of complications. Not to mention how emotionally difficult it was for me to put all of this on paper, because that called for me to re-live the whole experience again and again in my return visits to the many memories I'd tried so hard to suppress. There were many times I had to stop writing because I could barely see through my watery crying eyes. I'm not typically a crier—actually, far from it. All the surgeries, infections, cuts, digging for staples, needles, and everything between the sun and moon made me one tough motherfucker. Physical pain is not something I feel anymore. For example, I was just recently doing my daily routine of push-ups, and when I hit my max, thirty-five, I felt a terrible ripping feeling in my chest but decided to work through the pain. I managed to pump out another fifteen to make fifty and basically ripped all my muscles to the point of a small explosion in my skin and muscle fibers. The doctor was amazed that I was able to push myself past that pain threshold for that to even happen, but like I told you, physical pain is not really a factor anymore.

Emotional pain, however, is a whole other story!

I learned that life can really fuck with a person. This could be anything from getting diagnosed with cancer to losing a loved one unexpectedly to getting fired from your job. Any little curve ball can really screw things up. But so too can it make things amazing. That's the funny thing about life. It's very unpredictable and unforgiving. Just when you think you have it all figured out, all of a sudden, "Boom!" You have it so incredibly wrong and need to learn a whole new set of rules.

Think back to a time when you were let go from a job and the events that led up to it. Do you remember what you ate on that day? Or who you texted? What movie you watched that night? Probably not, because for that specific memory those details don't matter; for other memories, they might. I tell you all this with a request for your indulgence as I tell my story. Though some pieces may not seem relevant at the time, you must trust that they are, and that their relevance will be revealed in the future.

That's kind of how this book is laid out. I have so many memories and stories to tell, all of which connect in the broader picture. So if you get stuck on something, be patient—all will be revealed in the end. That's if I tell it correctly!

In the time between when I started writing this book and when I finished, I was forced to re-discover and solve one of life's biggest hurdles (regret) and a solution to something we will all have to face at some point in our lives.

But before I proceed any further, let me take a second to tell my kids what I wanted to tell them when we found out I was going to die:

Your road in life will a lot tougher than I ever imagined for you, You need to prepare for a lot harder life, much harder the path I am taking. You will be pushed to your limits with the hurdles you will have to face. You might be pushed to accept a new daddy, you will have to have someone else walk you down the isle. You might have to work summers and after school to help cover the daily bills that come with life. You will need to be a very tight knit family and need to support one another as this will equally as hard as it on you as it will be on the rest of the family. There will be many choices you will have to face and decisions of roads you want to follow , and this will define who you are and are going to be as a person . I need you to know my lessons in life and how they impacted me so you may have some added knowledge on what the outcome may be if you chose the wrong one. Kids this is my word of advice to help keep your relationship and bond together strong, please continue on with your Taekwondo, as nothing in life is more important than confidence in yourself. Martial arts will teach you discipline and confidence, and with this you should never have to live in fear, like I did. As you read on you will see how fear ruined so many things for me and caused me so many years of anger and regret. Fear and lack of confidence held me back from realizing my true potential, so there is no way in hell I will let that happen to you two. From my stories you will learn to live your lives in a way I would have hoped to be able to live mine: in fear of nothing and empowered!

Now with that said, please picture me sitting across from you at your favorite coffee shop, with my medium French vanilla, and let me share the story of my life and how I got to where I am today. To my kids reading this for the first time: prepare for some stories you've never heard about me and apply them in your lives as lessons about what *not* to do. To everyone else: sit back and enjoy this story about me and those key experiences of my life that revealed how dangerous the mind can truly become when your whole world changes in less than a few words—"You are terminal and will die in three months." I ask you,

What kind of thing would you be willing to do to provide for your wife and kids knowing that any and all long term consequences are off the table (like jail time)? For me I was getting the death sentence in 90 days or less if I agreed with it or not, and I didn't even do anything wrong. So if im stuck getting the death sentence anyway, I might as well do something and at least try to better the lives of the ones that rely on me and the ones I love. The question was what am I capable of pulling off and how am I going to do it so I don't at least get caught until after the 90 days is up.

CHAPTER 1

An Utter Disappointment

Though this is my complete story to date, I need be honest with you and tell you this is my second attempt at capturing it. Initially, my plan was to make a trilogy of books. In my first book, I would tell you stories about my life *before* I had cancer and how the cancer messed everything up for me. I would tell you how I found a lesion on my tongue and the multiple misdiagnoses that followed and how I strived to become a criminal. The second would be the truth of it all. And the third would be everything I am working on now. But after a few people read the rough draft of the first part of the trilogy for me, their view of me changed. They looked at me differently, and not in a good way. I had never considered the reaction I would get from the people who read my book, or how their view of me would shift. Had that been a consideration, I might have concluded that some people wouldn't agree with the decisions I've made. And that is exactly what *did* happen—even in spite of the fact that they were only reading a third of my story and had no sense of what it was building toward. Here's what happened:

When I completed the rough copy of the first of the books I'd envisioned, I printed it out and shared it with two people for whom I have lots of respect. These people—my mom's brother and a reporter

I'd met several months before when I was living in the Toronto area and was interviewed by him while I was helping out with the Arc 2 bunker—barely knew my story at all before they started to read what I wrote.

My moms' brother (who lived about four days' drive from me when I was growing up) only really knew of me what my mom told him. He only ever met me a handful of times in my life, but he knew I was struggling with cancer. For argument's sake, let's just say we didn't know anything about each other. Even before my tongue was removed, we never emailed or texted, let alone talked on the phone. All we had was a bloodline connection; otherwise, we were complete strangers. I only recently got in contact with him when I had to move across the country for my wife to go to school (to upgrade from a dental assistant to a dental hygienist), and my mom insisted we try to connect. It was only then that I learned he was an established author—hence why his opinion meant a lot to me. I was hoping he'd help me with structure and grammar, where I was lacking. After meeting him for the first time as an adult, I wished he'd not been so distant when I was growing up. He really is a nice and thoughtful man. Unfortunately (while not knowing it), asking him to help me out by reading my first book probably ruined any chance we had to connect in the future.

My reporter friend contacted me about four days after receiving the copy and told me he'd had to stop after reading about five chapters. In fact, he said if he were to continue reading, he would have had to call his lawyer, as he didn't want to put his family in any kind of legal binds.

My uncle did finish the rough copy of the book I gave him but called his lawyer right after. When I arrived at the meeting place, which was of course a posh coffee shop close to his house, he approached me with such anger and disappointment in his face. Seeing it was soul crushing for me and hurt more than when the doctor said I had only three months to live. At that moment, I was fully crushed.

You see, the first book explained why I was going to keep what I felt I deserved, the terrible things I was willing to do, and my twisted thoughts. To make my plan come to life, I needed everyone to know I'd committed a crime. So I had to write a book about a crime I committed. I believed this would sell—not because I'm such an amazing writer but because I was going to be the first person ever to publish a confession to a crime before anyone even knew a crime had been committed.

In both cases when I met up with them to get the book back and their opinions of it, I was surprised by their reactions. I had been expecting them to ask if I had actually committed this crime and what the hell I had been thinking. That *did* happen, in fact. But what I didn't expect was the expression of disappointment in their eyes.

Before the cancer, I was convinced that money was the most important thing in life because it dictates your position in our society. But when I got a second shot at life, I realized that what really matters is how you are remembered. Money doesn't go with you when you die, but we all crave it to feel powerful. We think it will make a huge difference. How wrong we are. I didn't want to pass away from some stupid complication from this disease without teaching my kids about this false assumption, without them knowing the *whole* story. If I died before finishing the second or third book, my kids would only know part of it. So that's why I decided to tell this as one big story. It's kind of funny how it wasn't even the words that were spoken to me from my uncle or reporter friend that changed my mind on my approach, but his look of utter disgust they both gave me.

You know that feeling you'd get as a kid when you did something so bad you thought your parents would kill you and you quivered in fear, but instead they told you how *disappointed* they were in you, and that felt worse? Well, that's the exact feeling I had when I shared my book at the start—and this from two people I barely knew. Before knowing the truth, they looked at me like I was a criminal who put them as risk just by reading what I wrote. I could tell they wanted nothing to do with me and that the sooner I was gone from their lives the better. The look in their eyes ripped out what I had left of my soul and crushed me.

Throughout our lives we're taught good from bad, but the truth is there *is* no good versus bad. There is only the perception you have of yourself and how other people see you. Just because someone accuses you of doing a bad thing doesn't mean you are a bad person. They might not know exactly why you did it. Also, things that are bad in one society might be perfectly acceptable in another. If you don't care about people's opinions of you or how you see yourself, the world is your oyster, and you can live without regrets. But if you are like me and were brought up with good morals and beliefs, the world can be a much harder place, and what people think of you really *does* matter. Because cancer changed my appearance and how I see myself, I was certain this would be a walk in the park. I am getting used to people making assumptions about me and being judged on my appearance, so I figured if people already stare at my deformed face and talk behind my back about the way I look and sound, nothing would change. Or so I thought.

I was wrong! There seemed to be so many different ways people would look at me—from *poor him* and *I'm glad that's not me* to *that is not a guy I could ever trust*. When I received the negative reactions from both of my test readers, I decided to not go through with the plan I'd spent quite a long time on. Being looked at like I was some sort of bad guy or criminal was not something I wanted to face, regardless of my shortened life expectancy. I wish they could have trusted me and known that, though I had to do *some* bad things, it was a necessary evil to be able to do so much good, but that wasn't going to happen. So with all my cards on the table, I knew that if I was going to do something to ensure my family's survival, I would have to make damn sure no one found out until long after I was dead.

CHAPTER 2

Knowing what rules can be bent

When I was told I was terminal, I lost all hope and knew I had to put all my focus on the only thing that mattered: my family's survival. Many years earlier at my first corporate job in the oil field, someone told me "you never become rich having a normal job". You might be able to sustain yourself and your family, but you will never be waiting for that one last paycheque to get deposited where you can say, "OK, *now* I am rich." Now that I knew I was to die soon, there was only one thought that continually haunted me: How will my family survive with my income about to cease, and is this something I can fix?

I knew I had to do something before I died, and that I had to do it fast, as time wasn't on my side. If I could figure out a way to fix this, I could not only secure my family's future but maybe also fix some regrets that had been tearing me up inside. So I worked on this plan for a long time and was close to completing it.. The final step to this plan was to have my book proofread by people I can trust—in my case, my uncle and reporter friend. I felt I could trust them to read it front to back and talking to me before reporting me to any legal authorities. That way, I could get their *real* take on it, as if they were just average people who didn't know anything about my past.

But before I could explain things, they dropped me like a bad habit. If only they'd stuck around long enough to hear what I had to tell them what would be revealed in the sequel to this novel.

The truth is, with my corporate background, I was able to find some simple loopholes in many businesses protocols, policies, and procedures. Typically most of these things are really irrelevant on their own, but manipulated in a strategic way , I knew there was something there. I knew I needed to go in a different direction (even though what I had planned would have worked had I not bolted from those looks of disappointment). So I started on my master-minding of the most secretive, elaborate plan ever, one that was so complex I literally had to write almost a whole other novel just to keep track of it. There was an unbelievable amount of things to track and follow , but if it was executed to the letter, I would be able to walk away with an unfathomable amount of wealth. I initially planned this operation to have a fall guy in case anything came back to me (while I was still alive). But as things progressed, I realized that if I did it correctly, I wouldn't even need a fall guy. If I could make it so there is no visible or provable crime, it doesn't matter what you admit to! I could tell the whole world I was a mastermind criminal, but without knowing the crime, there would be no way to prove I was telling the truth. You need to know what the crime was and when it took place, but with all the loopholes it would be possible to make it all vanish into nothingness. Yet what was left behind as a result was unfathomable.

My largest hurdle was that because I was doing this all on my own and behind my family's back, I was limited to my own thoughts. If I missed something, it wouldn't be like I had a team of people to help me figure it out. I needed to make sure I thought of every angle, from setting up fake email addresses to ensuring the things that were transferred or purchased included no trace of me. The fact that I was actually going to try to pull this off threw me for a moral loop.

But as time went by, I was able to close any and all loose ends. At last the day came when everything was said and done. I sat back in complete shock I'd been able to come up with a plan that was fully untraceable.

The only step left was for me to proceed with a test run. If I missed something, I didn't want to go to jail for life with no reward. So I tried it on a lower scale, where I had a couple of safety protocols in place to see if anything could be traced back to me or raised red flags.

Luckily I was able to test each thing on its own first to see if I was at all mistaken on what would happen. Once that was complete I just had to connect them all together and sit back and watch my masterpiece take shape and work for me. You know all those little loop holes that people can take advantage of if they want to bend the rules, I had figured out a way to shape the system to my advantage: Here's an example of one of these rules people bend, If you break something that you have been using for a while, and don't want to pay the price to replace it, you can buy a new one at the store, swap out the new one in the box with the old one, and return it for a full refund. You tell them it was broken when you opened it from the box. They take it back as if it was broken prior to when you opened it. Another example could be how if you mail a letter and "accidently " send it with out a stamp they will automatically return it to sender, anyone could swap their address to the shipping address and have the address of where you want the letter to go as the return address and mail it without a stamp. There are so many more loopholes, involving everything from supermarket points system (grey areas) to they way commissions to salespeople are paid out. If you can find how everything can work together, it isn't impossible to make money come from no-where, all it takes is a hell of a lot of time and dedication to connect all the dots, For myself though time was counting down fast, when it came to how many hours in a day I had free to work on something, I had nothing but time. With the medicine that was continuously pumped into me, it forced me to see things from all sorts of angles. If I was thinking of something one way from one persons perspective, the next time I reviewed it my mind would be in a whole other state and I would understand it from a different side or way of seeing how it worked. Kind of like how you would get two different reactions from people if you approached a situation in anger or with professionalism. I played out all situations in my head and worked out each reaction to each and every action. Most people don't know where to look for the mistakes in how companies are set up, but that was my expertise for over 2 decades, so why not use that to my advantage when I have limited time and there isnt any consequences for my actions. My 90 day countdown had already started so I had to either shit or get off the pot. I knew I had a good success rate of pulling this off because even if I had a deadline of 45 days at that 18 hours a days dedication. That would mean I would have almost 1000 hours into planning a perfect crime. They say it takes 10,000 hours to be a master at something, and with my 1Q of 146 I knew 1000 hours was more than enough time for me to get done what I needed to do.

If you followed me on Facebook you would have seen that I distributed silver coins across North America that were issued to me by the Canadian Mint, as that was one of my final test runs. I Didn't want to have any of those on my possession. Needless to say, I was quite happy when the test run was finished and a complete success!

When I came up with this plan, it was never to be written down in a book let alone even talked about with anyone. But as you read on, you will understand why my timeline not only forced me to write about this crime but made it 100% necessary for me to explain the actions I was willing to take. Anyway, as you know, I had to change my plan and opt to tell my whole story from the very first lessons to my current state.

But before we get to that I have to tell you what I have been through in my life, from incidents that happened before the cancer to things that happened after. If I didn't, you would never know how I got stuck in this position where I had to come forth and admit to this crime. This touches on what I found most important in my life as well as the lessons I learnt along the way.

CHAPTER 3

Second Chances

After years of battling tongue cancer, I seem to be coming out on the so-called winning side. Most people seem to think that because I was beaten down by this disease and survived, my life should be full of joy and light and I should appreciate every day of the rest of my life. Well, that just hasn't been the case for me personally, and though I cannot speak for everyone in my position, I feel I have a right to be really, really angry. One big thing that gets me so mad is that people just waste time like it's an unnecessary thing. Time is such a valuable commodity, and here is why I am so upset today.

I spent a lot of time thinking and soul searching and just needed to figure out what I wanted before I died. And as I said before, time is a commodity, so I wanted to make sure the time I took writing a book wasn't wasted. I needed to make sure my time at the laptop, hammering out my story, would be worth it. As far as I'm concerned, my story is not worth **writing**. So many people get cancer and so many survive and face the same issues that I face, its just I'm not sure how many normal people don't understand our struggles and how it affects the ones around us. Some people ask whether I feel guilty for living when so many others have not made it —I get that a lot—and the answer is, "Hell, NO!" Do I have a larger appreciation for life now that I've faced death and lived to tell about it? Yeah, of course I do. But nothing really to write about—or so I thought. I think people are always looking for my new outlook on life so they can compare it to how they live their lives. When this happens, and it happens a lot, I can honestly say it makes me feel a little heartbroken. It does that for two reasons. One has a little to do with my pride, and the other has to do with how people can behave, ignorant to the impact they have on people's lives. I found that even though they're acting like they're interested in whats going on with me, they're really only thinking of themselves. No one really cares about how I feel from day to day and the struggles I deal with—only the people who love me without judgment actually care.

Let's take my story for a minute. I am the only survivor/surviving participant from a group of people who were part of a clinical trial I was partaking in. People kept asking what was my secret to survive it, when really they should just be glad I *did* survive it, not *how.* They kept on, acting like there was some secret potion I took or a miracle cure I was keeping from other people. They always ask how I survived it in case they ever find themselves in my position. But, sorry to say, that's just not the case. There was no special thing I did. The trial is 100% the reason I'm still alive which I didn't realize it at the time, but there was a reason we were able to find and get on this trial, which will come later on. Though I'm sure others will say it was their prayers being answered, or the things my family made me do, I really do believe it was modern medicine that kept me alive—its not what brought me back to life, but it is what kept me alive.

I definitely *was* given another chance, and my personal spiritual experience *did* give me a new direction on life. I was on death's door and died a few times on the operating table, and I believe if anyone is to have a real experience with their maker, it would be the guy who has died and come back. My spirit back for a second chance at life and I have a very specific direction to follow.

Because of my own personal sense of pride, I didn't really want to tell everyone my life's story and how it led me to where I am today, because there are many things I am not proud of, and I don't want everyone to know about the awful things I have done. But I decided that I have to suck it up so that I can try to share a glimpse of how life looks through a dying man's eyes. Hell, maybe this information will help others see how they will want to live their lives moving forward, or how to fight to stay alive, or how to treat others in my position.

CHAPTER 4

In the blink of an eye

This disease changed how I will live the rest of my life, and how from now on I will doing what I feel will make my life matter in this world. My hope is that you learn from what I experienced, and be more prepared than I was, if this was ever to happen to you or a loved one.

Being able to come back from a terminal situation, makes you realize you have to soak in every moment and not take for granted what is right in front of you. You think twice about staring at your phone instead of spending the time with your kids and other loved ones. You realize that if you didn't have an electronic leash to someone who actually has no connection to you in your life, you would have had so many more memories with your genuine loved ones—and they with you. Maybe you would have actually finished that project you were working on, or got that thing done that you wanted to get done last year, or taken your wife out on a surprise date when you had the chance. Sadly, being terminal brought forth all the things I didn't like about my life . . . time that was wasted or things I did that I thought were important but really weren't worth the pot we piss in. Though my end goal was the same before and after cancer (support my family), the disease really opened my eyes to what my life had become and what supporting a family really entails. My morals shifted because of the cancer and the situation it put me in, but in the end, I will win at life and not let it slow me down! Everything that happened led me to figure out the most complex yet perfect crime of all time then made me switch direction to create a way for many others to keep their legacy alive, people just like you.

The intention of this novel wasn't to admit to any crime I was ready and willing to commit, but to tell my story and share some lessons with my kids and open their eyes about their dad and some of my regrets. You will learn a lot about my life and decisions I made and, of course, how things progressively forced me into planning the perfect, untraceable crime.

I started writing in the middle of my hardest struggles, about two years after I was told I only had three months to live. The day I was told that was one of the most horrible yet most eye-opening days of my life. In an instant, your perspective on life changes drastically. In the blink of an eye, things that mattered don't anymore, and things that you didn't think twice about (suddenly) become the most important things in your life. You are thrown into a literal life battle, regardless of your readiness for such a thing. And the same goes for all your loved ones. Their involvement is just as much a battle for them, as the battle you will face. But hopefully my story will help you see the struggles from both sides of the coin. This really explains how my battle affected so many of my loved ones, how this disease ripped us away from each other, and how it was necessary to ensure the survival of my family.

For me, being told I was terminal was horrific, devastating , and life stopping. But it didn't take much time to pass before I had a tremendous come-back-to-earth epiphany. My biggest realization was that I was not bound by traditional laws anymore. It didn't take long for me to realize that no matter the action I undertook, I had no long-term consequence to my action. And though that didn't change my usual day-to-day decisions, it sure changed my long-term goals. Now I had no long-term consequences what so ever because it was game over no matter what. But the biggest challenge I had to overcome was providing for my family, which was not something I could do over a long period of time like originally planned. My new goal was to figure out a way that my family could be happy and financially set without a provider husband or father—very do-able when you don't have to follow the typical rules of society!

Here is a scenario, so you kind of understand what I mean. Let's just say that the love of your life wanted more than anything to buy back her childhood house, but it was double the price you could ever afford and there was no way any bank would approve you for that much. It would be something you couldn't achieve for her because it was so out of reach. You would basically have to give up before you could even get started. But now let's throw in the curveball: "the diagnosis." You have been told without a shadow of a doubt that you will die within three months and there is nothing you can do about it. So what do you do with that information? Do you lie down and die or use it to your advantage?

Just like all things in life, there is good news that surrounds the bad—it's just how you choose to look at things. Yes, you will die way sooner than you ever thought, and most likely be forgotten over the generations to come. And no, you will not get to see your kids grow up, your daughter get married, or your son graduate and speak to his generation in a valedictorian speech. But here is the silver lining: no matter what you do from this day forward, you don't really have to answer for any of your actions. Now of course this is all within reason. But here is what you come to realize: anything you do that is against the law really won't matter because you won't be alive long enough to receive your punishment! With no real consequences to any of my actions, I figured: GAME ON!

CHAPTER 5

Never Give Up

You know that even if you were ever caught by the authorities, it would take over three months of paperwork, evidence collection and analysis, court meetings, and so on to process everything for a court case. And by the time everything was set for your sentencing, you would already be dead from your disease. With a terminal outcome (stage 4 cancer), and how it spread so much in such a short time, you know the final outcome is inevitable. Even if for some reason they fast-tracked your sentencing, as long as you were proud of what you did or happy with the result, what would be the big deal of living out the last couple of your dying days in a prison cell, knowing you'd done the right thing for your family? So with those new realities in place for you, could you figure out how to get her that house? Of course you could!

You could rob a bank, hold some kid for ransom, commit fraud, steal from ATM machines, take a golden statue from a church—really, with no conventional laws holding you back, you have many more options of what you can do to make this happen. (This right here is when my mom's brother knew he was not having any of this, he saw where this was heading.)

Well, this is kind of the basis of my thought process that led to what I did. In my story, there wasn't an old childhood house I was trying buy for my wife. In my story, what I wanted to do for my family was give them the financial support a father should provide for his family all through out their lives. In my upbringing, I was taught that a father/husband should financially support his family, no matter how humiliating it was to him. You can take pride in any work you do—it doesn't matter the job you are doing. The family supporter, regardless of their gender, must do what they must do to make the money to provide a roof over their heads and food on the table. Please note that I don't have a problem with wives working. In fact, I encourage it. It's just that I believe that the majority of this responsibility should be on the head provider of the family.

In my family, I took on the role of head of household, and I provided for everyone the best I could. But because of the diagnosis, I felt like I'd failed as a husband and in my role in the family, and that my wife and kids would now struggle for the rest of their lives. But before I talk about the plans I made to fix my problems and how they progressed into something that almost caused me to change my guiding principles, I first need to go back and tell you my story from the very beginning.

` I wrote down my story for two reasons. First, if I was to commit a crime, I didn't want people to think I was just some thief who stole to be greedy. I'm a good person who deserves what I feel is owed to me and my family, and the other is so my kids could know a little more about their dad and the lessons he learned over the course of his life.

Kids, through this book you will learn more about me before I was diagnosed with cancer and how I was as a father. I hope you will read about how things totally changed for me and what I now know are the priorities in my life. And I hope you learn from my experiences. Please remember me as your loving father and not as a bad man. Circumstances in my life pushed me in a few directions of which I'm not proud, but this was never the man I wanted to become—well, at least not until this point, but in the very near future. I will become better than the man I was planning on being.

For all of you reading this, I must take a minute to apologize for something that will happen from time to time throughout my story. I might get sidetracked and run on a bit. Most likely I will do this because you will need more of a backstory of how or why something may have happened, or where something is hidden.

But if you are to take anything from the story, I hope you realize that no matter the situation, no matter what, NEVER GIVE UP!

If you, the reader, have been diagnosed with cancer or any life-threatening disease or situation and picked up my story to figure out how to beat it, here is my best advice to you: never give up until the very last second of your very last breath! Make plans for the future and give yourself a reason to wake up every day. Give yourself goals to reach and projects to finish. When the mind is lost and not motivated to engage the body to work and fight through healthy eating and exercise, those muscles and your physical strength are lost. This doesn't help you recover. Those of you reading this with a loved one who isn't in the best of health—get out with them more. Do things together and make plans to help keep them active, both physically and mentally, to fight whatever they are going through. Just having friends show up and show support is everything. And not some stupid "get better" or "thinking of you" message on Facebook. An electronic message always feels more like you are a task on someone's list to-do list.

#1 Pick up milk.

#2 Pick up their kid from school.

#3 Text Dad that we miss him.

#4 Pull the ham out of the freezer.

Most of the time I wouldn't even remember who said it. I'd just remember some words because my name came up in a conversation, or someone saw a post on Facebook and felt they needed to write something so they could look the part of a caring friend. But for me, these things didn't boost me up or give me any ambition to get through this. The only people who helped were the ones who stuck with me and spent the time to show me I wasn't the only one dealing with life's struggles and that we would all make it through this as a team, because you need a team to be there to pick you up and motivate you to keep going. Spend some time with them, a few hours a week, or anything personal.

I had given up. But others who probably should have given up when all was lost, never did, and that's why I'm still alive today. So regardless of whether or not you think all hope is lost, never give up on yourself or others, because miracles happen every day and so do scientific advancements. You need to be at your best every day, even if all is lost, just in case that day is the day the miracle does come through. For me everything changed when a new immunotherapy trial came out. You never know—things literally happen every day.

Now for me, when people told me to fight and never give up the battle, I never knew what the actual fuck they were talking about. I'm sure that you don't really know what that means either, but I figured it out! I always thought: How the hell do I fight cancer? It's not like I could punch it in its stupid face! Cancer is an infection or a germ, not something I could physically attack But through many, many sleepless nights and a lot of bad days, I figured out (in my opinion) how to fight and beat cancer. The key was to stop thinking *I'm dying/poor me/I'm helpless.* STOP THAT. It's not just poor *you*, it's poor *all of us.* We are all affected by this shit disease. It's not only you who feels this horrible thing that's slowly or quickly draining you of life—it's also poor everyone else who loves you and has to see you suffer and just wants it all to go away. It's how they feel helpless and would, at a moment's notice, switch spots with you so you could live a happy, free life.

If you are so entrenched into feeling there is no hope, continue with that line of thought. But if you choose to do that, you better own it!!! You can't think *poor me* and *I'm going to die.* If you are going to go that route, man the fuck up and accept it!!!!! So even if you can't get out of that slump, don't go out like a little bitch. If you know you're going to die, make it count. Go out like a warrior. Give your family and friends the memory of you dying with honor and pride.

The key to your survival, be it physical or spiritual, is to keep making plans and living life, even if you gave up. You still have work to do! Let me explain: Whether it's making plans to go for a cup of tea with your mom or a friend, changing the brakes on your car or a friend's car, or just resigning yourself to taking a shower so you don't smell like a wet sock for when your wife snuggles up against you—make some fucking PLANS!!!

For me, I started off thinking: *I'm dying, and I can't believe this. Why did this happen to poor me?* Then I accepted it and owned it! That's really where my battle began. I started planning the MOST BAD-ASS, outrageous funeral of all time. On my deathbed, I was planning a funeral that would include a speech I had prepared in which I was going to tell off every last mother fucker that had wronged me. I was going to tell them *exactly* what I thought of them, where they went wrong in their lives, and, of course, how I saw them in my eyes.

On my death bed I was going out with a BANG—or so I was planning!

Most of the time you have two decisions in life: one that's right and one that's wrong. (Should I drink another beer before I drive home? Should I skip math class tomorrow? Should I lie to get away with something?) But on occasion , there is a middle option, or grey area, like the question of whether it's OK to steal bread for your starving family. This is an example of that middle area. For me, cancer stripped me of my life's goals and happiness. It ruined my future goals to give financial stability to my family and share my beliefs and life lessons with my children. I would have had a future with my kids had I not been poisoned with disease. So to make it right, I thought up and executed a plan to take back what had been taken from me. Let's call this "the middle area."

This book is my confession about how getting cancer almost turned me into something I wasn't, how I got a second chance at life to pass on my life's lessons and last words to my kids, and how I chose to spend my second chance fixing my regrets while delivering a gift to the world! If you are ready, Let's begin.

CHAPTER 6

Starting With a Kiss

I need to tell you all about my past so you can understand where I am today and where I am headed. When I was a young boy, I recall my dad coming home from work smelling like sawdust, like he did every day. My dad was a very hard-working carpenter. Back then, we did not have debit machines or bank cards, so finding money in the pockets of his work jacket or dirty jeans was pretty much guaranteed—and, boy, did I need to make a withdrawal. You see, there was this girl, Samantha, in my elementary school, and my gosh, she was perfect. The prettiest girl you had ever seen. And though she didn't know it yet, she needed to be my girlfriend. She had brown hair that was a little curly and the prettiest face, plus she was so kind and polite. Everything about her made me happy, and I had that puppy love we all so desire. She was the sweetest little person you had ever met. We were not in the same class in school, but we were in the same grade. She was in the French immersion program and I was in English, even though English was both our first language. Smart little cookie, she was. To impress her and get her attention, I knew I had to make a statement. And to do that, I needed some money.

Though I never made a habit of it, I went to my personal ATM machine—the pockets of Dad's work jeans! I never liked going through his pockets—not because it was a breach of his privacy, which I didn't care about (hell, I was just a kid), but because my dad always had Kleenex in his pockets, and I hated touching used Kleenex. Funny how Kleenex is now a necessity for me and how my kids will *always* get a handful of Kleenex when they reach into my pockets now (or step into my vehicle or sit next to me on my bed). Kleenex is now a part of me, because with no tongue, you must always have it on hand in case you decide to talk or open your mouth.

Getting back to the story, I got the money from his pockets and had a plan. I went to school as normal that day, but when that lunch recess bell rang, I bolted out of there on a kilometer-and-a-half run to a little convenience store called Peter Rabbits. Peter Rabbits always had beautiful fresh roses outside, and what girl could resist roses? No girl!! I had fewer than forty-five minutes to get there and back, which was difficult for two reasons: one was my little kid legs and the other was that you were not allowed to leave school grounds, which meant I had to be stealthy about it. Lunch was fifteen minutes, and then we had a forty-five-minute recess until classes started again. So the timer was on and this little guy was like a streak of lighting. I was running for love!!! I didn't even stop once!

I made it to the store, purchased a dozen roses, and was careful not to ruin them as I bolted back to my soon-to-be girlfriend!

When I arrived back at the school, I came up through the lower field, where all the kids played soccer. Just like most schools, we had our different groups of kids. We had the cool kids, the sports kids, the nerds. Oh, and we can't forget the socially awkward kids. I assume the girls had their own groups, but I never understood what they were. Who really understands girls, anyway? Lol. And then Samantha had her friends in a group I didn't know that well, because they were in the French area of the school and were divided into groups of their own. For the most part, the French and English kids didn't mingle.

So here I came all sweaty through the lower field with this massive bouquet of red roses for this girl I so desperately wanted to impress. As I started my way up the stairs from the lower field, my best friend (still to this day) noticed me with this bouquet and of course made a big deal of it. Next thing I knew, I had half the school (basically all the English side) following me up the stairs. Looking back, that climb for a little kid was like climbing the stairs of the Empire State Building—it just seemed to go on forever.

Anyway, I made it to the top and immediately started looking for Samantha. She usually hung around the same place and that day was no exception. There she was, looking so cute, and I was freaking nervous, like almost pee-my-pants nervous.

By this time, the whole school knew I had a dozen roses and that they were for Samantha. She walked up to me all red in the face and I handed her the flowers but with all these other kids surrounding us (which was by this point basically the whole school). They were like a bunch of elementary kids (which we all were) and they were all making kissing noises and stupid comments. So I didn't blame her at all when she just said, "Thank you," took the roses, and walked away.

Really, what the heck else was she supposed to do in a situation like that??? It wasn't my finest moment, but we're setting the stage for how things in my life don't necessarily work out the way I plan them. In this situation, I didn't even figure out the end game, as I was so focused on getting her some nice flowers. I didn't even think how it was going to go after she got them, and I definitely didn't count on the whole school watching. I had no real game plan, so her walking off was probably the best thing that could have happened at that moment. But life has a funny way of making things work out in the end.

At this point, everyone went back to what they were doing, except for my best friend. He just laughed at me for the remainder of the break—which, thank goodness, had only a couple minutes left in it until classes started again. I felt my plan blow up in my face, and my pride was more than hurt, but there was some good that came from putting myself out there. Yes, I was super embarrassed, but all hope wasn't lost, and this story doesn't end there.

We had another break later that day, and Samantha came up to me and took my hand and brought me to the center courtyard (this lush garden area in the middle of the school). And though I can't remember exactly what she said, it was basically that she hadn't thanked me the way she wanted to. And in this beautiful garden area was where I experienced my first kiss! Just Samantha and I, kissing in this garden, with all her friends watching and saying how romantic it was. A little awkward, but who cares? I got to kiss this amazing girl, and she was my first kiss!!!

From that point forward, Samantha and I were girlfriend and boyfriend, and she was the best thing since sliced bread. I remember riding my bike down this massive hill/street called Highlands Blvd. to her house almost every day just so I could see her. I usually overstayed my visits because I never wanted to leave, plus biking back up that hill was dreadful. She and I were great together, and I don't recall when or how we broke up, but maybe she will read this book and contact me and tell me what I did wrong. Knowing me, I probably did something really stupid. That's kind of my MO. But in the end, if I didn't put myself out there and take a risk, I would never have gotten to be as happy as I was back then. So take risks and put your self out there, because if you never take a bit of a leap into the unknown, that's exactly what it will become......the unknown.

CHAPTER 7

Fight or Flight

OK, this is very embarrassing, but I must tell this story, as it was a very important part of my life: the story of my first fight. I was in high school by this time, and you know how they say every person has a fight-or-flight reaction to times of high stress? Well, with regards to the flight option, what they don't tell you is that it should be called the so-scared-of-confrontation-that-you-chicken-out-and-don't-stand-up-for-yourself-and-regret-it-for-the-rest-of-your-life reaction. Because that's exactly the category this story falls into.

Paul (who was a really good friend of mine) and I went to Barb's house, where we were meeting up with her and Erin. Barb was a good friend of ours, as was Erin, and Paul really wanted to get to know Erin better. In fact, he was trying to hook up with Erin, and I was trying to get in the good books with Barb's little sister (sorry, Barb, but it was never you on my radar). When I say "little sister," it's not like I was super old—she was a year or two younger than us. So the plan, which is most guys' plan, was this: watch a movie, turn the lights low, and see what happens—again, there was no real end game to my plan.

Sadly for me , Barb's sister wasn't home yet that day when we arrived, but I knew she would be home after her gymnastics lesson, so we decided to rent a movie and see where the night took us. Back in my day, we didn't have Netflix or streaming. We had Blockbuster, which was where you went to rent a VHS. It was about a three-block walk to the movie place from Barb's house, so off we went—Barb, Erin, Paul, and I. Well, about two blocks into our walk there was a forested area next to the sidewalk, and two kids, probably about one or two years older than us, came up to us and basically said, "There's two of you guys and two of us guys, so let's fight." They were clearly drunk, which to me was unheard of, being that I was about fourteen and hadn't even thought about getting drunk yet.

There was a little guy and a big guy. Now when I say *little*, he was bigger than me, but he was little compared to the brute he was standing next to. They both rushed at us and Paul immediately got in the fighting stance. And I what did I do? I ran like a scared little chicken shit! (ARE YOU KIDDING ME???) I wish I could say I stood up for myself, but I didn't know how to act or what to do in a fight. I hadn't learned to hold my ground yet, let alone have the guts to confront a person who had full intentions of actually physically hurting me. So I ran like the wind!

Kids, that's why I am so proud of your taekwondo dedication. You both became black belts, and I know this will help with your confidence in life as well as your projection on the world. You both have turned into amazing little adults. I hope you will never have to experience the feeling I did in that situation.

As soon as I bolted, the littler guy chased after me. So on the spot I came up with a plan in which the one guy could chase after me, and Paul could either run or fight his guy. I didn't really have any other option as I already committed into running away. . But it didn't go that way at all. This was another time when things didn't work out as planned for me. I ran about half a block and the littler guy was on my heels, as I let him be. Maybe it was that he was drunk or out of shape, but I wasn't having to run too fast to stay ahead of him. When

I looked behind me, he was right there. So I looked forward and went about another block ahead. I kept my eyes forward, ensuring I didn't trip and get my ass beat because of a misstep. But what I didn't know was that he'd doubled back, so when I went the distance of one more block and looked back, there was Paul getting double-teamed by these two assholes. Besides the obvious beating he endured from these guys, Paul also got kicked directly in the eye, which instantly swelled it shut. It was some two weeks before he could finally open his eye and it was totally blood-red for about another two months. Luckily, there was not any permanent damage.

But here is the messed-up thing that Paul didn't know, that in fact no one knew: when the guy doubled back, I could have run back toward him to help out my buddy, but I didn't. I ran down the side road and around the block, not knowing what to do. I ended up helping push an old man up the hill in his wheelchair while my buddy was getting his ass kicked by two drunks. Paul, I will never forgive myself for not being man enough to take a beating to help out my friend. I am truly sorry.

After the fight, we all met back up at Barb's house, where I was enraged with anger because such a perfect day had been ruined so abruptly by someone else's actions. In fact, it not only ruined the day—it made an impact on my ability to trust people for the rest of my life. It also made me learn to always stick up for your friends whenever they needed it, regardless of whether they wanted it, and regardless how it may effect me mentally or physically.

I did eventually figure out who I thought it was that beat up my friend, and I reported him to the police. It was a guy who went to our school a few grades above us. They brought all of us into the police station, and while I was waiting to be brought in to identify the guy (I was the third person to pick him from a line-up out of us four), I said, "I hope they aren't just pulling up a yearbook photo."

Well, sadly, I was right. WTF??? That was it. They dropped the previous year's yearbook in front of me and asked me to pick him out. (Really?!?!? I guess at fourteen I was just as good a detective as they were.) No background checks into them or anything. I don't know what I really expected, but at fourteen, I thought I'd see fingerprints taken, interrogations, a real line up to choose from and of course reports filled out, not just some yearbook and a direction to "pick him out." I think I really was expecting more of a physical line-up of the criminals at large. The other three people said it wasn't him, but what I later figured out was that this crime was such small peanuts, they only went through this exercise to please our concerned parents. They didn't actually care about such a small thing. They would never really follow up on that—it was too insignificant for them to waste their time.

This was another lesson for me …. as this lesson applies to my perfect crime. If there is no way to prove you did the crime, or it doesn't get noticed, then there is no crime committed.

Oh, on a side note, two years later, I did get to kiss Barb's sister on my front doorstep, which my mom ended up interrupting by walking out the door at the wrong time . Thanks, Mom!

CHAPTER 8

Facing Your Fear

A few years went by and I started dating this girl named Emma who went to a different high school than me. She was a great girl and my first long-term, serious relationship. Things between us were going great until I ended it like a real douchebag. I have to tell you about a situation that happened with us before I tell you why I ended it, which is also why I feel like I deserve the cancer I got.

Emma and I met at my work, the PNE in Vancouver. I worked at the petting zoo as a poop picker-upper/maintenance guy, so this would have to have been around the summertime. I'm not sure the exact year, but it really doesn't matter. Not much to tell here except that she found this rugged young man very attractive and wanted to date me, so she told a friend who told me as much and, yup, that's how we started to go out! It was just that simple. The funny thing was that I never really noticed her at work because I never thought of work as a place where I was going to date anyone. I always acted like myself on the job, where people's real personalities tend to shine and they stand out as free-spirited individuals. So, kids, please always be yourselves and live your lives how you need to live them to be happy. Don't worry about how you might look in someone's eyes because, the truth is, if you don't care what they think, they will see you as someone amazing.

(And while you're at it, kids, find a job that you love doing, where you always wake up excited to see what the day will bring. If there is anything you don't like in your life [no matter what it is], put it out of your life for good. You should never have to wake up and hate how your life is or who you have become. Stay true to yourselves and live your lives in such a way that you laugh and smile and love freely every day with people you want to be around.)

Anyway, in this case, I *was* having fun and working hard and just being myself, entirely in the dark about the fact that that's what women actually find attractive. There are of course more requirements, like the person has to have a good-paying job, great hygiene, be fun to talk to and bond with, and, most importantly, be able to fix things around the house. But being yourself is the most important thing. So—some more advice—never feel awkward or nervous around anyone you find attractive. Be the people I raised you to be and show them who you really are … your beauty will shine like you couldn't imagine and they will be the ones that want to come to you!

In Emma's case, that's exactly what happened to me. I was being true to myself and giving off *my vibe*, and she was digging it! I never really noticed her at work prior to the initial approach, but you can't really blame me. We did work at a petting farm where we had to wear a uniform of fluorescent green T-shirts with white collars and dark jogging pants while we scooped up goat, cow, sheep, and rabbit poo. It wasn't really an attractive job to work in, so needless to say I didn't see the diamond in the rough initially. But thankfully she had the courage to say, "Hey, I'm right here and I think it's worth seeing if we make a good match!" She really was a diamond in the rough, I just needed her to to point it out to me , as I was blinded by the job I was there to do

Back in my day, that's typically how people met. We didn't have a swipe-right option or an autobiography you could consult online prior to seeing if your personalities were going to mesh, like "I'm a funny, well-spoken individual who likes horror movies and sitting by the fire at night." I don't need you to tell me how I will see you: You're not a funny person until you make me laugh. You're a well-spoken individual by whose standards? Is your family from the southern States or some remote cult, and are you are the first one in it to mask your Southern drawl? You might be a person who yells at movies as if the characters in the film are going to talk back to you. Or maybe your definition of sitting by the fire isn't the same as mine. Maybe you go out with a dozen of your friends every weekend to have a huge raging pallet bonfire complete with draining a bottle of vodka and telling rambling stories about your kids, who never talk to you anymore.

For me personally, there's something to be said for picking who you want to spend your time with as opposed to just going off what the person has written about themselves and how they imagine others see them. I'm a funny person—but *are* you? I'm well-spoken—if you compare me to a guy who has no tongue. I like horrors (we all know it's a bad idea to look under the bed, but thanks for embarrassing the shit out of me). I like "sitting by the fire." We all have to make decisions about whether we could be compatible with other people, and I prefer the old-fashioned way that involves mystery and wonder— which makes me want to tell you how my beautiful wife and I met, and I will … but later in my story.

So things were going well between Emma and I, and she was so nice and sweet to me. Really, she was better than a diamond in the rough. She was a precious gem that only I had, and she only had eyes for me, like I was the perfect man for her. If we weren't together, we were talking for hours every day on the phone. Then one day she told me about this boy who kept teasing her and was just being a complete asshole to her at school. I knew that if this continued, I would have to do something about it, as I was not going to let the same kind of regret fall over me as when I didn't stick up to those guys when I was with Paul. I knew she would also see me in a different light if I didn't do what was right. So a couple of days of this went on and the day came when it was just too much for her; she was just in tears. She called me when I was at school (you know, on my flip phone ... I was super bad-ass!) and told me how this guy (if I'm remembering correctly) pushed her into a wall and was calling her names and starting rumors. Well, I was outraged that someone would do this to anyone, let alone someone I cared about, and I had to protect her. So I and two of my best friends jumped into my car (a 1988 Trans Am that we nicknamed "the chicken" because of the massive blue firebird sticker on the hood) and off we went to her school across town to kick some ass!

We arrived at her school and walked in like we owned the place. I have to add that my friends came with me not because they had my back—which, if it came down to it, I know they did—but more to watch me in my first real fight and see me get my ass beat down before they jumped in and took care of business.

Well, as I mentioned before, this was going to be my first real fight. There was no way I was going to back down, regardless of how big the guy was or how many friends were with him. I was prepared to take my beating because sometimes in life you have no other option but to do what you know is right, notwithstanding that you don't know the outcome. So here I was in a school full of people I didn't know, randomly walking the halls looking for ... who knows what? This was the first time I had been into her school, but I wasn't in there thirty seconds before I saw her, and this guy was literally shoving her around, pushing her in the halls while people were just ignoring what was happening around them. Well, a protective instinct kicked in and all I could think was: *You're going to fucking*

THE DANGEROUS MIND OF A DYING MAN

die, mother fucker! The "That's my girl, and I will protect her at all costs" attitude kicked in, and I stepped between them and was all set to throw down. Shit was about to hit the mother-fucking fan!

I squared off like I was ready to throw the first punch, and I knew I was going to throw a bunch of hell fire punches to his face regardless of whether he took me down. I needed him to have a bloody face just to prove I wasn't a person that would let this kind of thing happen, regardless the outcome. Hell, I would have bitten his ear off just like Tyson in the Holyfield fight, but what happened next I would have never guessed in a million years.

This guy, who had a good foot on me and probably an extra six-inch reach, started to cry like a three-year-old who had lost his blankie. *WTF, was he actually crying right in front of me when I was clearly a much lesser opponent?* That just made me feel like I was even more powerful, and, in the moment, I didn't care that he was crying, because for what he did, he still deserved a straight-up ass kicking. But he wouldn't *stop* crying, and eventually he turned and ran off. The good thing was that I looked like a hero to my girl, but, more importantly, after that incident he never did anything to her again. And to this day, I have never had a one-on-one fight ... not yet, anyway!

Now, as promised, I will tell you how we broke up and why. Sadly, I am so ashamed of my actions here. I would like to say it was mutual, that it was overdue, and/or that it was for a good reason. But, sadly, it wasn't, and I am a selfish asshole, and ashamed of my actions. I don't want to go into details, as it's not fair to her or anyone else in her life, so let's just say her mom had cancer and was very sick. Like a coward, I jumped ship to avoid the stress that was to come. I couldn't handle it. I tried, but I wasn't a strong enough man. I was just a kid, and it was too much for me to handle. Please don't sympathize with me for the decisions I made here, as I was truly the villain in this part of the story. This was when she needed me the most, even if just for moral support, but I was not enough of a man and I left. I never even gave her a reason why; I just said I'm sorry but it's over and drove off, leaving her crying on the side of the road in front of her house. I not only let her down in her time of need, but I let myself down. Imagine how hard it was for her seeing her mom deal with the effects of cancer, and the only bright thing to your day decides to abandon you and not even tell you why. I am a real piece of shit for doing this and regret it every day

Kids (Zack and Kisenya), if you are reading this for the first time, here is where you *must* learn from my mistakes. Just because things look to be difficult, do not bail like I did. I promise you will regret it for the rest of your life, and it will probably be something you will never be able to fix. Would the relationship have lasted? Probably not. Your first long-term relationship doesn't typically last. But don't leave it because things look like they will be hard. That's why you have us (your parents). If anything ever gets too hard, come to us and we will always help direct you on the right path and pick up any of the pieces you accidently drop along the way. I promise you, you don't want something like that hanging over you for the rest of your life. And, Emma, I need you to know I am truly sorry for being a selfish shit and that you didn't do anything wrong, and definitely didn't deserve what I did to you. It was 100% me being a little boy and not a man.

CHAPTER 9

The Game Changer

To everyone reading this, if I can pass anything on from my experience with cancer, almost dying, and getting a second chance at life, it would be not to let someone else's selfless actions destroy a love between two people. In my case, I'm talking about the love between a father and son. Love is really the only thing that matters in life, but that can be ruined by evil. I will tell you how I learned this lesson and how it was the hardest lesson I learned in my life—all because I couldn't come to terms with something that happened to me over twenty years ago. This thing that happened was fully outside of my control, but this situation caused me one of the greatest life regrets, one from which I will never really recover. It happened close to the end of my high school years.

When this incident occurred, it tore my life apart. It was such a senseless crime that had been committed against me (destruction of personal property), but it was something that literally ripped apart a child's bond with a father. I do hold a specific person responsible for this, and I will make this right for me personally/mentally. But this experience with my life altering twist of survival taught me that it's never too late to come forward and express your feelings to repair the love between two people—as in my case, the love between father and son.

When I was lying in my hospital bed, my biggest regret was that I didn't do something to ruin his life as he ruined mine! I will tell you all about it and my plans moving forward.

In my original manuscript, I had this asshole's name written in the book, but my editor said I had to remove it because of potential lawsuits. She said I was not allowed to threaten a person even if I had changed their name in my story. So I need to be careful how I word things as I don't want him to think I was ever threatening him in any way;

She also said something that caught me off guard. She said, "Forgiveness is at the very core of Christianity," and my writing about this individual completely contradicts core values. My response is simple: Finding God or discovering a higher being is completely life-changing, but it doesn't change who you are or how you feel towards things overnight. It's not like you find God or your epiphany or happiness and everything changes with the snap of a finger. The truth is, my life-changing experience revealed that there is another level to life, and I connected with my maker in a way that I will never really be able to explain. But just having that experience once doesn't change a person's deep values and feelings. It's not like people go to church once and say, "I found God and I know everything that's required of me and how I should project myself onto others." The truth is, people go every week to learn how to be better or see things in different ways. I know over time and through my interactions with life from a different perspective that I will find forgiveness, but as for now, at the time of this writing, I'm still not quite there yet. There was a lot of hatred and anger built up around this one specific incident that happened to me, and I am going to tell you about it. I just need to leave his name out of it or call him another name to keep his identity private (according to the editor).

So let's call this individual (Malady). I know it's an odd name to pick , especially for someone that was convicted as an accomplice to murder back in 2011, but if you spend the time to look up the meaning behind the word, it will totally make sense on why I picked it. Let me start by saying, "Fuck you, Malady". In my life's story you represent everything wrong in this world and in my life. Way before I was even diagnosed with cancer, you were the cancer in my life that I couldn't shake.

Like with any good story, this one has a good guy, who has all the odds stacked against him, and an evil that lurks around every corner. And in my story, I like to think of myself as someone who has good morals, opposed to the piece of shit you turned out to be. If that upsets you Malady I apologise, but my readers need to know the kind of person you are. Now, for my story, I didn't actually need to bring that up from your past to remind people of the kind of person you are, but I like to be thorough. Kids just between us (I hope my book makes it out for the world to read so people can figure out who I am talking about and re-surface his past, and I hope all that darkness returns back in his life.)

Malady, when you choked me out in the computer room, you embarrassed me and belittled me. But see what happens when you cross people… They never forget what you did to them, and one day they come back to get you. But not me, I would never do anything to harm you;)But today is the day I say enough is enough. Kids, this is a lesson to always remember the people who disrespect you. Never forget who did you wrong or lied to you, take your time and get back at them when it best fits your schedule. Don't act on impulse, act with intelligence. Now here for my story with this individual. What he did caused me and my dad to lose what should have been an un-breakable bond. I should have fought you over 20 years ago, but because you were too chicken shit to come forth and admit what you did to me, because you hid and lied about your involvement, I was never to have this more-than-deserved fist fight—what would have been my first real fight. But time passed and because you never came forward, too many years later I found out that you were 100% involved in the incident.

Knowing what I know now, if we were to actually throw down, even your own mother wouldn't be able to recognise you when I would be done with you. But that would never happen because I only intend to talk to you at our schools 30th reunion in the middle of the football field......Say 8pm?

Malady, I hope your identity is never brought public for your sake, but I have to add you as you are a big part of my life and drive to live. Let me start by saying

Malady, when I was at my weakest, one of my only goals was to outlive you just so I could piss all over your grave. I know that may seem way over the top, but you need to understand that (at the time) that's about all I could really do to stand up for myself and my pride. I didn't want to take the pain of not doing something about him, back to the grave me for a second time. But unfortunately with the limited strength I had left, this was the only thing I could see me being physically able to do, to stick up for myself. I had to rely on my wife or kids just to help me up the stairs. The worst pain of it all was having to see the hope in my wife's eyes slowly die as she watched the love of her life wither away to nothingness. Anger was all I had left and I decided to use that get me through each day.

I made a promise to myself that I was going to battle every step of the way and have goals, and my most realistic /achievable goal for a pain I was living with all my life was to outlive the guy that wronged me to piss on his grave. That was one of the first goals I had that started me on my uphill battle. I was making goals and setting deadlines for things that I needed to do to keep me driving forward, Even if I was too weak one day, I would schedule something that forced me to get stronger. For me to be able to piss on your grave, I needed to keep living through each day so I could outlive you. Miracles happen every day, and who knew, maybe the next day I would see your name in the obituaries and have that chance to fulfill that life goal, which (to be honest), looking back, seems pretty fucking bad-ass to me! As for you, Malady, if you are man enough to show up to our reunion in 2027, I will not piss on your grave when you die. In fact, I will call the matter over with, as we will get a chance to "talk" when I see you at the next reunion.

On a side note, if one of the family members of the boy's body that you allegedly helped dispose of wants to talk to you , then I will gladly step aside for them to chat with you .

So, what did this individual do to me that makes me so mad you ask? Though he never did fess up and act like a man, Malady, I know for a fact that you and your friends were the ones that vandalized my dad's 68 Dodge charger (the exact same car that my parents used when they were dating) You destroyed his car beyond repair, and destroyed our family . This car, my dad handed down to me as my first car, which my dad and I restored back to full running order together. I was literally less than a couple of days away from handing the keys back to my dad after so many years of restoration, and share that moment with him, but I was never able to fulfill that dream because you stole it from me. Maybe one day I will get the chance to find him one from the same year and the same color, though it could never be the exact same 1968 Dodge Charger he owned, because you destroyed it beyond repair. Realistically, that's a memory I will never have as even if I could replace it it wouldn't be the same car with the same history, and instead I only have your aftermath. So I'm going to take something from you right now, your dignity!

To learn what this guy *really* took from me, you need to know my relationship with my dad and family and some of our background. For those of you who don't know, my dad is the most amazing dad any kid could have. He's a carpenter who worked his ass off to get us everything he could. My mom also worked her ass off as a very hardworking banker and full-time mom. My parents both worked hard all their lives to give my sister and I lives they could be proud of. It makes me laugh to know my dad literally had to write his marriage proposal to my mom on a piece of paper when they both worked cross shifts and he couldn't stay awake long enough to even propose to the love of his life. He felt it would be best to write my future mother a romantic note asking her to marry him, as he just couldn't wait any longer but had to work.

There was so much love when we were kids, and though our upbringing was not perfect, it was perfect for us. I am so proud of both my parents and the job they did raising two amazing kids. Jenn ✓ (my sister), the one who never gives up, is now a big-time movie set designer/purchaser and owner of an exclusive gin company called Copper Penny. She was the best sister a younger brother could ask for—yes, we fought like a typical older sister and younger brother fight, but that was natural, as she always wanted to be the one in charge because she was older, and I thought I should be in charge because I was the second man of the house. Jenn, I know I always joke that I am the favorite, but, honestly, you are the better kid. Because of my decision to move away at an early age, I started my own family far away and wasn't around when I was really needed while Mom was going through he battle with cancer. Jenn, you were the one that was with Mom every day. I have never seen someone more dedicated to their family, career, and friends than you. You win! You are always there for our parents. I was the one who moved away; and now that I'm a loving parent, I see how horrible that must have been on both our parents with my selfish act.

Growing up, we would go on family bike rides and play tennis or just hang out. There was this one time my dad had asked the guys he works with (when he worked up in Whistler) to shovel as much snow as they could into the back of his truck so that when he got

42

home from the job site, having been gone for so many days, his kids could play in a truck bed full of snow on a hot summer's day. We still have the pictures of us literally dressed up in full winter gear having a snowball fight in 25-degree summer weather!

I also remember the times when my dad would put me on his lap and I would steer the truck while he was in control of the gas pedal. I do that with both my kids now which I know is a special memory we will always share. So, yeah, my dad and I were close; we had such an amazing bond and friendship with each other.

All that was completely destroyed because of that guy and his friends/associates back in what I believe was in the year of 1996. You can reference that story in the *North Shore News* in North Vancouver.

For those of you who don't know cars, the car at the heart of this incident looks just like the car in the *Dukes of Hazzard* car, , orange and everything. It was built a year before the Dukes' car. The main difference was that the 1968 model had round taillights, and the '69 one had rectangular taillights. That car now goes for about US$68,000—but that one was priceless to me. What hurt the most was that I was never going to be able to give my dad that moment

This guy not only smashed in the windows, kicked in the sides of the car, cut the white leather interior, bent the fucking wiper blades and antenna, and kicked in the flip-up grill that covers the lights, but he shit on my life's dream of giving my dad his first car back, fully restored. No, he literally squatted in the back seat and took a hot, steamy dump of human waste on what was years of building this specific connection and bond with my dad. After all we did together and the bond we had, once this happened, it destroyed me inside and killed my soul. After that, I could never really face my dad. It's not like my dad ever blamed me, but still to this day I can't look at him directly in the eyes for even a short period of time. My mom told me in secret how badly that affected my dad and said she'd seen him crying. My dad didn't even cry at his mom's funeral—not because he didn't love her, but because he was taught not to show emotion for people to see—so knowing that this brought my father to tears fucking destroyed me. I kind of hope once this book hits the public eye and your past resurfaces, we will both have a vendetta to fulfill. The question you need to ask yourself is: Am I willing to show my face and have the world know who I am and stand up for my actions?

Because I know I sure would like to talk to you.

The bad thing for you is when it comes to my story almost all people will side with me because I am the good guy between the two of us and also the underdog. If you decide not to show up, we will all know that you are not only guilty, but also the very definition of a coward. If you do show up and get the talking to of a life time, no one will actually give a fuck about you, because they know you are an actual bad guy, regardless of what you do or say from this point!

Of course, there is the possibility you might show up and beat me up, but that's probably unlikely because I am going to spend the next eight years dedicating my life to learning how to crush an opponent. But in the rare case that happens, everyone will hate you and you will be known as the murdering asshole that beat up a cancer victim. Funny how things can go so badly for you in just one day. As each day ended your past was another day forgot, and now look what I did, I brought it all back up. You had over twenty years to man up and confess what you did to me, but now, no matter what, it's a lose-lose situation for you. If I lose or win, I still get to look back on the day as a great one that helped try to fix something that went wrong in my life and how I chose to use my second chance in life to fix one of the worst choices I made that, to this day, still tears me apart inside. So, kids, sometimes in life people will say it's not worth it and to just walk away, but sometimes you need to know if it could possibly be a life-changing decision that you will regret for the rest of your life. If so, don't listen to that one person or one voice in your head that says to just walk away from it, because sometimes in life walking away is not an option!

You might ask yourself how I found ot that it was for sure him, well guess what Malady, your sister came up to me at a house party all wasted and high and while laughing, said, "I can't believe you haven't figured it out yet that it was my brother and his friends that totally fucked up your car." I always suspected it was you, because you chased me down in the school to say "It wasn't me." And that was hours before I even knew the car had been vandalized. You destroyed it over the weekend, and I had yet to make it down to the school's mechanic shop to see what happened. And here he was squirming like a little bitch, trying to lie his way out of trouble. I never had proof, but your sister ratting you out, was exactly what I needed to know who and where to direct that anger.

I wish I could say my dad and I were always close regardless of that, but after that there was always that awkwardness/separation I couldn't repair.

On my death bed when I faced the heavenly gates, which I am told happened a few times, God laid out a path for me and continuously gives me advice and updates on how to spread His gift to the world. But even with that all happening around me, I won't forget what you did to me and my family.

I will repair the connection with my dad, and I fucking damn well will restore the honor you stole from us. I will give you one chance to properly apologize for what you did and replace what you destroyed. If you choose not to do that, I wont waste any more time with you and instead I will go back to my original plan of just out living you. Then I will make sure to have a dog shit on your grave, just like you did to me when you shit in my car. If you decide to show up and face me like a man, then I will call the matter over with and wont disrupt your plot. Its funny how I bad I just made it for you , your past has been brought back to the fore front for all your family and friends to remember about you, which is pay back for choking me out in the class room, and I get you stuck in a catch 22 where if you show up everyone will know what you did to me and hate you, and if you don't come you know there will be shit where your final resting place is. What choice are you going to make?

OK, that was a lot more info than was necessary, but once I got started on the subject, it brought up a lot of old feelings. Anyway, I feel like this is a little self-healing I needed to get to. It's been bottled up and stirring up a lot of anger for so long!!!!!

CHAPTER 10

How The Grad Prank Started

Now for the final lesson before I get into how life led me to where I am today. This lesson is to never assume something—either you know or you don't. If you were to sum up my high school scene (and I hope I'm not dating myself here), I and my group of friends would have been like Greasers in a school full of Socs.

The high school I went to was aimed a lot more toward business and computers and a lot less toward blue-collar jobs. Because I wanted to be a mechanic, the teachers had no problem asking me to fix their cars and do their brakes, but they never returned the favor. They never spent the time teaching me beyond the school parameters to help me better myself. I learned that no one besides your true inner circle will ever just volunteer this to you. In life, if you ever need any help from someone or need something to happen, you make it happen by demanding what is owed to you or speaking up for what you need. Just because *you* may see the whole picture in your head, others may not. So if you are struggling with something, always bring it up to someone you love or trust and ask for help. As for me, I expected the teachers to just *know* what I needed help with. I put my trust in a system that's flawed. In life, you need to fight for every inch. Don't just expect people to do their jobs correctly or help you out. For me, because I didn't ask, they would never help. So instead of learning the traditional academic life skills, I learned ... other life skills. Many times I ended up spending school hours behind the school racing my Trans Am ... which was always an easy win because the rich kids usually bought Honda Civics or Camaros that had V-6 engines to save on gas—LOL. Wannabes.

Believe it or not, kids, there was a time when a cop pulled up next to me and challenged me to a race just to see if he had what it took to beat me. After I beat him, I was shocked when he wrote me a warning ticket that said "Race with a police vehicle." He had challenged me! I asked him why he pulled such a chicken-shit move of pulling me over when he was clearly enticed by the race, revving his engine at a red light and challenging me, and he said, "Well, I was already behind you, so I figured I would pull you over and see what you had under the hood." We had a good laugh about that and went our separate ways.

Your time in school (for all students) is such an important developmental part of your life. This is where you make life-long connections and face so many obstacles. Some things you may run from and some you may stand your ground on. But your battle in school and how you become the best person you can be is an ongoing one because you will be presented with new challenges by the day. School is like your life's training simulator. And, as with any training simulator, it's there for you as a learning tool. You are free to stop at any point and ask for help, because this is your only practice shot before taking on life head on! As long as I am alive, kids, I am here to help you learn and grow. Never forget that the people with whom you associate will determine the kind of person you grow into.

The group of friends I hung out with were loyal to each other and helped each other. They still do, though I have been pretty distant since moving away and distancing myself. We were the only ones to do any grad pranks in our graduating year. They typically ended with the cops showing up. Which brings me up one particular prank—one that went so wrong so quickly.

This grad prank we concocted over a few drinks and a few minutes was, we thought, the *perfect* grad prank. In truth, we didn't put that much thought into it, but it involved our borrowing all the baseball wire fencing (which was stored in a container at the local park), transporting it to school with my buddy's car and trailer, and then surrounding the school with it and locking everyone out the next day. It wasn't very well thought out, but hey, we were kids being kids. We got the fence to the school and that's about as far as that plan went. But before I continue, I have to tell you this next story, as it explains why I was going to be in a world of shit.

CHAPTER 11

Don't Smoke The Profits

Two days from this writing, pot will be legal across Canada—but back when I was in high school, it definitely was not. So here is how I became known to my classmates (for a short while) as a drug dealer. The drug we are talking about, kids, is the same one that's going to be sold in local stores, the same one your mom insists was a contributing factor in what saved my life. We are talking about marijuana, also known as pot or weed.

When I was about seven, my mom (your grandmother) told me, "Jason, you are a little different from most kids. If you ever do any drugs, you will die." She said anything from the doctor was OK, but if I did any other kind of street drug, my body would shut down and die. So, believing everything my mom said as truth, I took that at face value. DRUGS = DEATH.

Later in life when I was working at the PNE and sweeping up goat and other petting farm animals' poo, I noticed a rolled-up piece of paper on the ground. Knowing damn well what it was, yet never having seen a real-life joint before, I picked it up and stashed it in my pocket. After work, I went home and hid it in my room. About three months went by and I was hanging out with a good friend of mine—your uncle, let's call him Robert—talking about what girls' groups to invade next, and he pulled a bottle of rum from behind his TV and said, "Let's get wasted tonight!" Because I never did like the taste of alcohol, I had a moment of stupidity. I ran home, grabbed the joint, and said, "You drink that, and I will smoke this!" Now don't forget, I had found this on the ground and didn't know anything of its origin.

We walked to the park and, well, to make a long story short, it did what it was supposed to do. I was so freaking high I thought I was floating. I laughed for hours and hours. In fact, it lasted a lot longer than I ever expected. I felt like I wasn't even real, so that was the end of that! No more doing that again, I said, although I was laughing at the time because I knew I wasn't really there. Between us, I was not a fan of that!

About four months later, I was talking to a friend about that experience and he said it was probably laced with something like cocaine or some sort of acid. I then realized that if I could have a moment of weakness like that, knowing that if I had any drug I would die, then anyone could have a momentary lapse of judgment.

The reason it came up in the conversation was because my group of friends had decided they were going to buy some weed for the weekend. I asked where they were going to buy it and they said off a guy whose number they'd gotten from the stall of the bathroom. Right then I knew I had to do something, because if my friends were getting into it, then it was a trend that would go around the whole school as it was the next hurdle in life we were all going to face. But how do I fix /stop what they are so hell bent in doing? I spent some time thinking and came up with a solution. If I couldn't stop the process, I could streamline it and make it better. You see, it wasn't that they were going to smoke pot that worried me. It was that they were going to buy it from someone they didn't know, and I didn't want them to have some sort of overdose because they bought some shit laced with seriously dangerous drugs. So I did my research and found a guy who grew his own pot locally. I made a deal with him to buy his weed. The only stipulation was that I had to be there during the cutting process—that way I would know nothing was added to it. Because I knew I couldn't stop what was happening, I would supply what I knew to be "safe" to people in my circle.

Call me paranoid or call me a guy who takes the opportunity to make money when it presents itself, but the fact was I knew that the people around me were going to get what they wanted with nothing extra added. This also solved the problem of my not having to tell the guys that I didn't like it when everyone was doing it. You know that peer pressure everyone talks about? Well, that was also a dilemma … and this fixed that. If I sold it, why would I smoke my profit away?

I wanted to be that guy who could stand up for himself and just say no to drugs, but I didn't have the confidence against group mentality. It may not have been the perfect solution, but it was what I thought was best at the time.

I sold weed to my inner circle of friends for about six months, until the thrill of smoking it died down—which couldn't have come quickly enough, because a man who was about thirty acting like a new student came up to me in school and asked to buy a marijuana cigarette. Seriously, who the hell calls it that. My instincts kicked in and I realized someone had ratted me out—which, I have to say, was probably a great thing, as I could have easily gone down the wrong road if I'd stayed with it.

When the thirty-year-old approached me, of course I said he had the wrong guy and went to class like nothing had happened. But later in the day, I grabbed everything I had and flushed it down the toilet in the school washroom. To be honest, I can't remember the last time I have been so relieved. Finally, that whole thing was over with and I could go back to having a normal life without people showing up at my house at all hours of the night or sneaking into my back yard to ask for weed, nor did I have to worry if today was the day I would get caught.

Kids, here is another lesson I want you to remember: never be a damn sheep. Always do what you know is best for you. Don't just do anything because other kids are doing it or because your friends want you to. If they are *real* friends, they might try to push you a bit to see where your boundaries are, but in the end, if they are a true friend, they will respect your decision. If they don't, that's a key indicator that they will be a poison to you later in life, and my suggestion is to cut all ties with them. Sadly, some people you will meet in life will try to persuade you to do things you don't want to or that you know are wrong. To be honest, it's always a little scary to stick up for yourself, because no one likes being singled out as *that person*, but if you don't stick up for yourself and hold your ground, who else besides you is going to do it?

Remember a few years ago when fidget spinners were popular, and everyone had them and we laughed at all the kids who followed the crowd? Well, same idea. I want you to be able to think for yourselves, and I never want you to be a sheep! As we said, people are either sheep, wolves, or sheepdogs. The sheep are basically the followers, the wolves are the bullies, and the sheepdogs are the ones who protect their pack. Kids, I have been training you all your lives to be sheepdogs, so stand up for yourself and for the ones you love, especially when you know they need it. The ones who earned your love also earned your support and respect, as it's a two-way street. If you see your friend struggling with a problem, be it at school or home, here is where you learn who you are as a person. Will you stand up for them, or act like nothing happened? This is something you will come across many times in your lives, so you need to decide how you want to live your life, because it's 100% up to you.

CHAPTER 12

How the Grad Prank Finished

Continuing on with the grad prank story ... the cops showed up at the school when we were off-loading the fencing, I'm sure the people in the houses by the high school were just concerned with what we were doing so called the police to check it out.

Well, when my buddy yelled, "Cops, run!!!" that was exactly what I did! I dropped what I was doing and, like a panicked Olympian, bolted the hell out of there. I didn't realize that no one else actually ran. When the cop car stopped, one of the cops jumped out and chased me on foot! No one else from the group ran, and if I had just stayed put, nothing would have happened, because I was in a group of about twenty kids. The two police would have just told us to put it back and smarten up. But no, I ran off because I had weed in my pockets. I ran down the side of the school and ditched the weed in a bush. I obviously wasn't going to head back towards the police, so I continued running toward the backstreet round-about. Still not knowing about the policeman who had jumped out after me, I stopped to catch my breath and, as I looked back, saw a hand reaching out from a man in a full-out sprint. His hand must not have been more than six inches from me when I immediately blasted off in a full-on adrenalin rush.

The back street ended about fifty meters from me, where there was a massive stairwell down a hill and back up the other side— probably about 200 stairs down and 200 back up. Well, I'm down and up the other side in 5.6 seconds flat. I bet you I broke the world record for running from the cop on a down- and uphill stair race. He chased me for a while but ran out of breath—*have another donut, Copper*, I thought to myself, not realizing that they carry a ton of gear on them. I assume it's probably hard to run with an extra thirty pounds of things strapped to your chest, plus he could have shot at me at any time if he'd wanted to.

Because I had run from the group and abandoned my only means of getting home, I walked to my friend's house, about half an hour away. I had a cigarette while waiting for him and he showed up about halfway through it. He told me what happened after I ran off. He said the cop who was chasing me went back to my buddy, who had stayed with his car. The cop grabbed him and slammed him against the wall, and then the cop punched the wall next to his face. He demanded he tell him my name. Well, my buddy always had my back and knew the bro code and to never be a rat, right? Wrong. He sang like a freaking canary: His name is Jason Kom-Tong; he lives at 3 50 5th Ave., 90090, his phone number is 415-561-4900, he has a sister named Jennifer, his mom's name is ___ and his dad is ___. He owns a dog, he likes vanilla ice cream, his social insurance number is 427055273, and so on. Thanks for that, Paul (one of my best friends that I trust so much). Thanks a lot.

Learning this kind of knocked me down a peg from thinking I had won the game of cops and robbers. Now I knew I had lost—and lost bad. Lol.

A couple of hours passed, and I headed home when everything had calmed down. I very quietly came in the front door, knowing everyone should be asleep, but what did I see lurking in the dark, sitting up waiting for me, but my mom. OH SHIT!! In a very calm manner, she said to me, "Constable Smithsonian wants you to call him back right now. Here is his number." *For fuck's sake! I was a dead man.*

I called the officer and, like I suspected, he was a complete douche bag. "If I had caught you, do you know what I would have done to you boy?" he asked. So I said, "But you *couldn't* catch me ..." (Yeah, not the time to be cocky.) But he very politely and calmly responded to me: "You had better make damn sure I don't *ever* catch you, because I will make you pay for making me run after you."

The obvious lesson here? DO NOT GET CAUGHT if you're going to do something bad. Or if you do something bad, bring it forth before you get caught. It's better to ask for forgiveness without the chase than to ask for mercy from one pissed-off person who had to waste precious time trying to find you. Or, better yet, if you must do something bad, keep that secret to yourself so no one can ever say it was you who did it. That was my plan for supporting our family. I was never going to tell any of you what I did.

CHAPTER 13

My First Big Choice as a Man

This experience happened the day of my eighteenth birthday, while I was standing in the army recruitment line. The recruitment office line was in the armories building a couple blocks from the house in which I grew up. I always knew as a kid that I wanted to protect the ones I loved, and the best way I knew to do this at the time was to join the military. They would give me the skills and knowledge I needed to protect my loved ones. It was the same reason I joined ✓the air cadets—the 103 Thunderbird Squadron—when I was a kid. My experiences and the lessons I learned with them enforced my conviction that joining the military was what I wanted to do with my life. Protect our country and our people as best we can if needed , and give everything to that cause , which was my life. I was willing to truly die for what I believed in.

Many people on my mom's side of the family were in the military. All but one of her brothers fought in the Vietnam war. Sadly, I don't know many of the stories. Maybe my uncles didn't want to re-live the horrors they'd seen, or maybe it was too sad a story to tell their nephew—either way, I can assure you I was not influenced by my family to join, not in the slightest. The topic never really came up, because I never told them it was something I wanted to do. I knew if I did, my parents would tell me no.

The armory was also where I attended air cadets, where I learned discipline, respect, and, of course, friendship. But what the cadets also taught me, though I didn't realize it at the time, was that there is a system to everything—rules that must be followed to make things run smoothly and to maintain order, no matter if you are in the military or the workforce.

I learned that people, for the most part, lust after direction and rules to follow. Even the person who chooses to be a drug dealer (who everyone looks down on) follows rules, though they may be different from those you follow. We all follow a pattern or system. We all have morals and a code of ethics we choose to follow—we just may see things in a different light or through the experiences we've had in life. Some people are just trying to scrape by to the next payday, and others' biggest concern is they can't decide what boat to buy.

So there I was, waiting in the military recruit line, and all I could think about was my mom's voice and facial expression when I got home and told her I'd joined the real military. Always in the back of my mind I knew what the right choice was. But at that moment, I was making the first real, important choice I could make as a man. And instead of doing what I wanted to do with my life, I made a man's choice and did what I knew was best.

I reached the front of the line, and the military recruitment soldier looked me in the eye and said, "You're up next, son."

I thought, *Maybe I am making a huge mistake. I should talk with my parents and not just make a move without their blessing.* Besides, it's not like that was the last day the military recruited people, and if I spent the time to talk it out with them, maybe I would get their blessing, which is really what I knew I was missing and needing for a life-altering decision like this one.

So in a moment of shame while looking into the recruiter's eyes, I turned around and walked out of the line-up and to my Trans Am and drove away. To everyone there I must have looked like a freaking coward, and I'm sure they all had a good laugh. But I was so very relieved, not because I walked out and didn't join, but for giving myself a second chance to talk to my parents and get their blessing, which, unfortunately, never happened—not because they said no, but because I never brought it up with them. I didn't want to show my cowardly face to the recruiter again, and I didn't want to tell them how close I actually came to being recruited to train for some war I didn't actually know anything about. Though I do feel like I may have missed my calling, I don't regret my decision. Sometimes, other people's feelings matter more than yours.

You will know this when you find true love. But in the meantime, you can fully trust those people you have let into your inner circle. These are the ones who would never intentionally steer you wrong. If I was to join the military, it would have broken my mom's heart, not so much for the action I did but for the act of making a choice that affected everyone I knew without considering them or giving them a voice. Such complete trust is a powerful weapon. You can use it for love, leverage, or complete evil. I will write about a fellow named Guy, who was purely evil, and how I warned people of his character the instant they met him.

I always knew I had more important things to do in my life than just live day to day. I was meant for something much, much bigger— I just didn't know it would be this. I was sure it was supposed to be a military thing.

On a side note, since the cancer diagnosis, I have tried to join the military over the last four years, but they will not accept me because of my disability. Really, I lost a piece of skin (my tongue) I just want to do anything I can to help protect people, especially now. But now I know my purpose in life.

CHAPTER 14

Dont Run From Your Problems

Living with the guilt of what had happened with regards to the car, I was not able to face my dad anymore. I felt like I had let him down. That was the biggest factor behind my decision to move to Alberta. I told myself that I would work in the oilfield and grow into a man. But the truth of it was that I was not able to deal with the situation that happened to me; I ran from my problems.

Kids, if I am able to teach you anything in life, it's that you don't run from a problem. Stand your ground and fix it. Sadly, I learned this the hard way, and I don't want you guys to ever have to experience that. Now, that being said, please don't mix that message up and think I regret how things turned out, because that's just not true. Just because I may have moved to Alberta for the wrong reason doesn't mean I would change a thing if I had a chance to do it all over again. I wouldn't even give it a second thought. Because of those choices I was able to meet your mom, fall in love, and finally know what true love really was. And, of course, we can't forget the best thing that ever happened to me, which was getting the privilege to be your dad!! I would do it all over again, again and again, just to have you guys in my life! So, kids, here is the story of why and how

I ended up moving to Red Deer and how and why you were raised in Alberta.

When I moved to Red Deer from North Vancouver, BC, I was dating this girl named Sandy, and she was OK, but I should have known from the day we met that she was not for me. But hey, I'm a guy, and I hadn't learned that girls can be evil—not yet. By that point in my life, I was only very critical of myself and didn't think that others had it in them to be evil ... so here is the story. Sorry, Sandy, but you were the poison in my life out of all the people who cared about me. This is what can happen if you don't listen to your family and friends when they tell you someone's there for all the wrong reasons. I was blind to what they saw, but if I'd actually taken a step back, I could have easily seen this.

I had a party at my parents' house, which was one cool house for parties. Upon opening the main door, you entered through double doors that the previous owner had glazed in a light lacquer. You took your first step into the grand entrance and immediately smelled the newly lit spiced-apple-scented potpourri. If you turned to your left, you could walk the long hall to the end, where you would reach the large living room that had an open view of all of Vancouver. From there, you could turn left and go toward the bathroom, my dad's office, and my parents' room. If you turned right, you had the option of going into the kitchen (which also had an amazing view of the entire city and a bird's-eye view of the backyard pool) or the formal dining room, which connected with the open living room. You could also go straight to a stairwell that led to my man cave.

If you went down the stairs, it would take you to a door that opened into a huge open space. In this space there was a very large, fully stocked bar, a wood-burning fireplace, and way off in the corner, the door to my bedroom. My room was the only one in the house that wasn't updated ... except for the yellow carpet. Yes, a puke-yellow carpet. How gross. My room didn't have charm, but all

I ever needed was a basic room. I'm a boy, and as long as I could sleep in it, what the hell did I care? So this large party space I mentioned had a glass door that opened to this not-too-big-yet-not-too-small swimming pool. (When my parents went away for a weekend or on a small trip, I would crank that pool up to hot-tub temperature and doggy paddle around naked. I'm sure the neighbors saw my bare ass a time or two, but it's a nice ass, so who cares! :)

The party started quite early as parties go, and people came and went all through the day. Sandy was no exception. She came with a mutual friend of ours, stayed for a bit, and left. The sad thing for her, or the first warning sign I should have picked up on, was that I didn't even notice that she was there at all. So when I got a call from a friend saying that this girl who had been there thought I was attractive, which I definitely was, I was too embarrassed to say I didn't even know who she was talking about. I lied and said I did, and she asked if I thought she was pretty, which, because of my first lie, meant I had to tell another to cover my ass. So I said yes, I thought she was pretty. This turned into: If I thought she was pretty, would I want to go a date with her? At that point, I found myself stuck in my own Catch-22. If I told her I didn't want to, she would want to know why, and I would have to tell her that I had lied and had no idea who she was talking about. Or I could have just played out the lie and gone on a completely blind date. Hell, I was even wondering if my friend was just messing with me and there wasn't a girl at all.

Needless to say, I said, "For sure, I want to take her out on a date." Besides, getting a date wasn't a bad thing at all. It wasn't that I was desperate … I was just lazy, lol. So I got her number and address, which was on E. Nasa Parkway, and I headed out a couple of days later to meet this girl, and I didn't have a freaking clue what she looked like.

I got to her apartment building and knocked on her door, then this girl answers the door and … wow! Is she ever good looking! I was thinking to myself, *How the hell did I not notice her? She is really sexy!* Then she says, "You must be here for my roommate!" Oh, yeah, I guess so. Damn it ... lol.

So the girl was OK, nothing too special, quite plain almost like an albino, but I was single and so was she, so it made sense. We went out on our date and, honestly, I don't remember how it was. I assume it was just one of those first dates most people have. We dated for quite a while and decided to move to Red Deer, Alberta together. It had been my idea. I wanted to move there to work on the rigs and make mad cash. Plus, I had to avoid my dad at all costs because of the guilt I felt. I had been staying at Sandy's apartment for the previous six months to avoid my home and the guilt I felt on a daily basis, so I figured I could move away and bring my girlfriend with me because I knew we lived well together, and I trusted her. She said yes, and she had a few friends in Red Deer and wanted to come with me.

I don't recall how this all happened, but I ended up going there first, finding and getting settled into a small apartment with the idea that she would come up a week later. I would love to hear her side of this part of the story, but what happened for me opened my eyes to how hurt you can get if you let the wrong person into your life. I didn't hear from her for about three days, and then she showed up at the apartment, dropped her stuff off, and went out with her friends. After, she called to say she would be spending the night at her friend's—and she never came back. She called me up a couple of days later and asked me to send her stuff and said she was moving in with some guy. I think we had been dating for about three years at this point. What the actual French fry???

So obviously I didn't know what the hell was going on, but she wanted me to mail her things. I had just moved to Red Deer and didn't know a soul in that foreign town. I did meet the landlord's son while moving into the apartment, but he was only there because he was stealing my light bulb to smoke crack out of it. Maybe she left because she saw that small, shitty apartment. I guess I may never know.

With her out of the picture, it was just me and Jessie, my dog— but that was OK. If I was to prove myself as a man, this would be my starting point! I got a job right away at the local meat-processing plant, where if you had two feet and a heartbeat, you were guaranteed a job!

I became friends at the plant with a guy named Jarod. He's in jail now, but he's a real nice guy, just made some bad choices. I quit that job after about a week, as did Jarod a week after me, and I got a job working for a hydro vac company, where I met the boss's niece. She instantly took a liking to me and wanted to take me out and show me around Red Deer, which was really great, as I didn't know anything about the city. The boss was the one who introduced us and encouraged her to take me out and show me around. But when the boss saw how much time I was spending with her, he assumed I must be sleeping with her, so he fired me. I wasn't I swear! And fuck him for even thinking that. She was recently separated and had a newborn, so there was no way I was getting caught up in that soap opera.

Needless to say, it was a bad day for me, having been fired that morning, so I went to my apartment and sat down for a beer or three—Kokanees, of course. Halfway through my first beer, my buzzer rang. I was thinking, *Who the hell can this be?* I looked to my side and, yeah, Jessie was at my side, and I knew Jarod was out of town on a well-testing oilfield job, and that was everyone I knew in Red Deer. Except for one other person Sandy

I answered the buzzer and guess who it was. The ex-girlfriend's new boyfriend, there for her stuff. At that point, I figured my new start at life had beaten me down enough and I was going to fight back. This guy was the first step.

I asked him, "What the hell do you want?"

He said, "I'm here for her stuff, and I'm not leaving without it!"

I told him, "You can try, but as I told her, she's free to get it at any time, but there's no fucking way I'm giving it to some asshole that comes to my door threatening me."

At this point, I knew it was time to stand my ground and I buzzed him up to my second-floor apartment. I grabbed the trusty baseball bat I kept at the front door, walked to the top of the entrance stairs, and looked down at him at the bottom. The guy looked like a freaking linebacker.

"Come on, motherfucker," I yelled down to him. "Come and get what you came here for!" With this, I held the bat in a full-on swinging position. He looked up at me on those stairs and said, "Well, she sure isn't worth this," and walked out.

A small victory! Turned out any man with some drive and the balls to hold his ground really *can* pave his own path.

CHAPTER 15

Tricked Into A Career

I wasn't in Red Deer long before I got a job as an oilfield well tester, same as my friend Jarod. Really, I like to think I was tricked into this career, because I actually applied just to prove a point. I really didn't expect to get the job. In fact, it was just a joke, but funny how things can just happen in your favor. One day while driving around town killing time and smoking cigarettes, Jarod turned to me and said, "There is no way you could become a well tester. Well testers not only have to be strong, but they have to be some of the smartest guys of the oil field. It's not about brawn with them; it's all about brain." So because I had my huge duffle bag full of the stuff you needed to work the oil field that I'd purchased when I moved to work the rigs (you know, fire-resistant coveralls, a hard hat, green king gloves, steel-toed boots, winter gear, etc.), I drove to the most sought-after well-testing company, parked my truck, and went in with my rig bag as a joke to see if I could get the job. I walked straight into the manager's office, threw my duffle bag on his desk (which made an explosion of paperwork and pens), and stood tall in front of him, puffing my chest. "I'm ready to go to work," I said in a firm voice.

He instantly stopped what he was doing and gave me a look like he was going to fly over his desk and tear my head from my throat.

But what he said totally shocked me: "Then don't just stand here—go see the secretary and fill out the paperwork. You start in twenty minutes. Also, get your fucking bag off my desk!"

I got the job…..WTF?!?!

So a few years went by and I was all about the oilfield life, working my ass off and totally loving my job. Everything was going perfectly—up until I met this guy named Guy.

CHAPTER 16

Some People Are Poison

Guy was one of those write-off losers you're amazed has made it this far in life. One of those slithery, snake-like people. And there I was stuck with this asshat for over three months in the middle of the Northwest Territories, freezing my ass off in minus-35, and all I wanted to do was get back to the comfort of my apartment. The one-month job turned into a three-month job, because that's just how it goes in the oil field sometimes—one day you're told one thing and the next you're told another. So it wasn't unexpected when they called me and said my relief was not going to come up because they'd quit the night before. Though not unexpected, it still pissed me off, because I hated working with sleaze ball Guy. But I liked the pay, so I stuck it out like I always did!

I know the proper pecking order to follow in a company—you respect it like you would in the military. Though you may not respect the person, you must respect the position. Well, that sums up the working relationship Guy and I had. I always had to cover for him and fix his multiple mistakes and mend the fractiousness between him and the company men on a daily basis. I will never jeopardize the job or my financial stability, so if I had to go above and beyond a couple of times—or multiple time, as with this scenario—then I would suck it up and be a man. But this didn't mean I couldn't hate this man on a daily basis.

I hated this guy—and I mean to the fullest. For one, he was dangerous to work with. To give an example, when we first arrived on location, he tried to spot the unit backward—literally, backward—so I knew right away this was going to be a very long job. It didn't take too long for me to fully take over while keeping him in his acting role of day supervisor. I spent all my time ensuring the job was done perfectly, which made him look good.

A couple of months into it, I found out through one of our consultants that our company was going to be offering a helicopter job. The job was to work in remote locations way up in northern Alberta, flying all over the northern forests in a helicopter all spring, summer, and fall, ensuring the wells were flowing properly. It was the perfect job for me. Plus, they had a cabin at the helipad where I would live with my dog as a home away from home. The company was looking for the best well testers to become battery operators, and they were going to train and pay for their helicopter licenses and supply them with a helicopter for work ... perfect.

All Guy had to do was say that I was doing all the reports and I was running the job and doing all the repairing and correcting and that I was the one that was actually running the job. He could have told them it was me who checked on the other company's crew when I saw what looked to be the wrong color of smoke coming from their flare stack, and that it was also me who stayed and safely shut down all the abandoned equipment I found running when that crew walked away over a money dispute. He could have said I was the one who had saved them millions of dollars and public humiliation, which would have caused a huge drop in their stock price. He could have said that all that was me, and that I didn't once ask for recognition because I knew better than to go above a supervisor to look good. Guy had a choice to make. Would he be the sheepdog looking out for his own and step up and say, "I think the man you need to be talking to is Jason"? Or would he take a less moral road?

I found out later he went with the latter and got the interview. And while he eventually also got the job offer, he failed the hiring process due to testing positive for drugs in his system. But that's his story, not mine!

I was just finishing up a very long three-month job on my birth-day, which happens to be on St. Patrick's Day, so the crew and I went for some drinks, which turned out to be a lot of drinks. We had a few in us when, later that evening en route to the next pub, Guy stopped the truck to go buy another pack of smokes. During this time, and I have no idea why, Guy turned to me and yelled, "You fucking dumb Chink!!!" right into my face. Well, normally I just let things roll off my back, because when it comes from a lesser man, what did I care? But that wasn't going to fly now that the job was over. You see, this act of aggression directly in my face questioned my authority in front of my crew. I had no choice but to confront him. If I hadn't, I would have committed company respect suicide. There are times you have no choice but to stand up to evil and what's right. Always try communicating things through, as violence is always a last resort, kids! But just remember, it *is* a resort you can utilize if need be, so don't be scared to stand up for what's right in this world. The choices you make today are the memories you will have to live with. The question is: What kind of person do you want to be for the rest of your life?

I sat in the truck for about a minute, waiting for my anger to settle, but it didn't. So I stepped out and walked into the gas station convenience store and stood directly between the ATM and Guy. He was pulling cash out for his smokes. I could hear his money being dispensed while I stood there.

"I am giving you this one chance to retract that statement and apologize," I said. He replied by laughing in my face. So I took one step forward and, with all my might, slammed both my hands into his chest. He fell backward into a potato chip rack, which exploded the chips all over the place. I was surprised how far I'd shoved him and looked right away at the man behind the counter. I very politely asked him to call me a cab, as I knew if the police showed up I would be thrown into the drunk tank for sure.

I headed for the door and there was a taxi there as soon as I walked outside, which I assume took me about thirty seconds. Now looking back, the taxi was probably already there, and the guy was probably calling the cops. But for now, I like to think he ignored what had happened in his store and called me a cab. The taxi driver took me back to my hotel, where I decided that, because it was my birthday, I wasn't going to let this idiot ruin my night. So I continued to drink by myself in my hotel's pub, which happened to be a strip bar on the weekends. I knew the next day was an easy one because all we had to do was head back to home base, drop off the equipment, and finally come home again. So, I proceeded to drink at the strip bar.

It's not uncommon to be put up in a hotel/strip club combo, either because most oil companies picked the cheapest hotels (for cost reasons, obviously), or the town was so small that it would be the only hotel around for miles. Usually, we had a job come up last minute and the managers had to scramble to find a hotel to house the staff. On this occasion, it had been a financial decision. The company didn't like spending money and that was OK with me, because I was alone. Who really cared what kind of crappy hotel I slept in?

So I was drinking in the club, which sat about twenty people. It was a really small place, the kind of bar you could tell was just hurting for any kind of customers. On that night, they had two girls who would dance their three songs, take a break, and dance again. It was one dance an hour, I think. Anyway, this girl was dancing on stage and she kept looking at me whenever I would turn around from facing the bar. Now don't think I don't like the naked body, because I do, but I was still so damn mad from earlier that all I wanted to do was get drunk and wait for the next day to come.

A few songs later, the dancer came over and sat on the stool next to me and started talking to me. She asked why I looked so upset, and we had a really nice conversation. It started off with typical stuff, like "How you are tonight?" and I said, "I'm just glad the day is over and can't wait until tomorrow." You know, typical small talk. But as time went on, it got more fun, like I was talking to a buddy. There were times our conversation was interrupted because she would have to go on stage and dance, but we would pick up where we'd left off when she sat back down. Each time she got up to dance, I never did watch.

Prior to her last dance of the night, which she was readying to perform for the five people left in the bar half an hour until last call, I was still feeling perfectly sober, though I knew I had a ton of drinks in me. (I knew my new friend wasn't drunk at all because I had been buying her milk all night. She told me she didn't drink when she was at work.) She asked me why I had chosen not to watch her dance, and I looked her right in the eye and said, "How could I? I know you now, and that wouldn't be right." She got a little offended and said that because I knew her, that was more the reason to watch her. She said she expressed herself through the beauty of dance and move-ment and that she really wanted me to watch her last performance because she was going to dance just for me. She said she was going to lock eyes and dance just for me. Not going to lie—it was one of the sexiest things I have ever heard.

She later went on to tell me she had many directions to go in life, and though she had the option to go to university or college, she'd decided this was the best route to get the money she needed to do what she wanted. Funny how I didn't think of that as being an option; I just figured life had beaten her down, not that she'd wanted and enjoyed this profession and took pride in her skills.

The bar closed at 2:00 a.m., and, like I said before, I was feeling sober … but only until I stood up! I was actually so drunk I couldn't stand up. I literally had to hold on to the bar stool to be somewhat vertical. At this point, I thought, *Hey, it's 2:00 a.m. This must be the perfect time to call my boss and tell him what happened with Guy.* I also wanted to tell him all about this wonderful experience I had with Guy for the last three months.

Now take a second and imagine you are a manager of an oilfield service company and you are at home with your wife or husband and you get a work call at two in the morning. Any sane person would automatically think, *Holy crap, this must be an emergency, not my drunk employee calling to tell me how he hates working with his co-worker.* In my mind, I was thinking he had better get my side of the story before Guy's. But in all reality, I should have waited until I calmed down and sobered up! It's funny because, even though I knew talking to him at that moment was a bad idea, I still wouldn't shut up or hang up the phone. Surprisingly, I didn't get fired over this. But if I had been in his position, I for sure would have fired me, lol.

After that, I went to the washroom, and stared in the mirror with the stupid look thinking to myself , Yup, I way over did it this time. I made it up to my floor where my room was and could barely read the room numbers while dragging my face across the hotel walls trying to get to my door. After that, all I remember is waking up in my bed, fully clothed and wondering, *What the actual fuck?*

Well, it turned out that the maids had opened my door the next morning and dragged my sorry drunk ass onto the bed. They knew it was my room because I was there for the last three months. I knew that Guy and I had a plan to travel in a convoy back to home base, but after what I did to him in front of our crew members, I knew he would be long gone. He was supposed to pull the flare stack while I pulled the office trailer and we would all travel together, but just as I suspected, he had taken off without me, which I was totally OK with.

I knew I had had too much to drink that night, but I was trying to figure out what had actually happened, and why the hotel staff were laughing at me. Had I fallen asleep outside of my room without going in like they were telling me? Well, I figured it out when I was locked out of my room from trying to get back into it after breakfast. The magnetic key card I was using had a different picture on it from the one I'd been using for the last three months. I was using someone else's key! Then it all made sense. The dancer must have slipped me her room key, and I had been trying to use it to get into my room. So stupid! So with that all figured out, all I had to do was go home. But that turned out to be harder than I thought!

Because of my own actions the previous night, I was feeling like absolute garbage. I knew it wasn't the best choice to leave when I was planning on leaving, so I called home and let them know I would be leaving four hours later. I didn't feel drunk, but I wanted to make sure I was not making a poor choice. All I had to do was the nine-hour drive back and I would be done this job. Check-out time rolled around at the hotel and I hopped in the truck and off I went. I came up to the last stop sign in town and was going to make that last turn before the straight shot home. I saw this car coming up from my left with its right turn signal on. It started to slow down to make the right turn, and I started to pull out. And guess what happened. The driver sped back up and kept going straight. The next thing I heard was BANG! Because I was pulling an office trailer, once I commit-ted, I was fucked. There was no strategic maneuvering I could have pulled off in that short period of time.

She drove right at my driver's side door and plowed her car under the running boards of my truck. She lifted the driver's side off the ground by about three feet. She then backed up from under the truck to put my truck back on four wheels. I was fine, as was my passenger (my helper), except that he had also watched the situation as it played out and, full of adrenalin, jumped out to fight the driver. Little did he know she looked like a ninety-five-year-old grandma. We instantly calmed down and the little old lady laughed it off like it happened all the time. I called the police, as her car, for all intents and purposes, was not roadworthy. My truck had a large dent in the door, but nothing I couldn't easily pop back out if we decided not to run it through a repair shop.

I handed her my license to switch info and she held it close and far from her face, trying to focus on it. At last she said, "Just tell me your name and address." The lady was basically driving blind.

On a side note: When is our government ever going to fix that????? Why isn't there a mandatory driving test every ten years, or five years??? Just my opinion.

Not long after that the police showed up and asked who'd called it in. I told them it had been me and asked them to talk to the little old lady sitting in her car. She said she had been going to turn and had decided at the last second to continue going straight. She said she didn't see me pull out, but her vision was not what it used to be. I was totally OK with—she'd told it the same way I had. But then, totally out of nowhere, the cop wrote me a freaking ticket for not yielding to oncoming traffic. Umm ... what the fuck?!?!? I was the one who had called the cops, and she had said she was in the wrong. I now had to pay a penalty on top of the hassle of all the paperwork and phone calls? That just triggered a switch and made me blow a fuse. So the accident aside, now I was pissed for being blamed for what was clearly not my fault. It would not only put a mark on my perfect working record, but it would take money away from my family that I'd worked so hard to earn. I turned to the cop and said, "Dude, seriously? What the fuck?" The cop just said the rules are the

75

rules, regardless of who is in the right or the wrong. So being hung over and just pissed off in general, in the most belligerent manner I could, I told him, "Fine, I'm going to drive up to the next intersection, throw my signal on, and ram the next motherfucker I see as hard as I can, and you can't do shit about it."

What this cop said next was priceless. He stopped what he was doing, looked me in the eye, took a breath, and said, "If you do, I guess he will get a ticket too!"

That completely caught me off guard and I laughed the whole way home. I had to answer for the truck and, yes, I got in shit over it. But that enforcement officer had such a great way of turning around the heated moment and defusing it with only his words. What it also showed me was how insignificant flaws are in all sorts of things that still must be done or enforced. I was thinking that my ticket was just a ticket, an insignificant piece of paper that gets processed through a system that is fed thousands of tickets a day. My ticket, which said "Not yielding to oncoming traffic," is the only documentation of the situation, and it will get buried as something insignificant. Funny how one little thing can completely change your whole day, or even your whole outlook on things. Since then, I have been noticing little flaws in every system and recording them. But what I really got out of the situation was that people can be assholes to you, but it doesn't mean you need see it the same way as them and ruin your day. Sometimes you just need to roll with things that are out of your control.

More time passed, and Guy was accused of doing drugs on location. He called up that oil company and took the job that should have been offered to me and failed the pre-employment drug test—idiot! And as for me, they promoted me into a day supervisor position, which I had definitely earned. I had put my time in and learned the entire job, inside out, to ensure I would be the next one to move up. Believe it or not, kids, I was a hard-working guy who would do everything to get the job done and done correctly. My job and work ethic was the thing I was most proud of. Much like my dancing friend from the bar, I wanted to do what I loved doing. Being in charge while thousands of pounds of pressure of highly explosive gas surged through a solid pressure-treated heavy metal pipe that you just installed hours before, while it ripped through and around the information room, filled with data-driven manual valves and levers, was incredible. That rush, knowing there is a pressurized pocket of gas kilometers deep into the earth's crust, and that you are in control. And all while there is a flame so high it's lighting up miles upon miles of land. During the night when we did our routine mandatory checks, we didn't even need a flashlight. Picture that: knowing it's 2:00 a.m. and it should be pitch black outside, but it's so bright it's just like an explosion on the surface of the sun when a burst of inner gasses explodes out of its core. And I am right there, controlling the power of the planet. That's how I saw my job and, as I'm sure you can tell, I loved it. Better still, I could make the money to do what I wanted in life.

CHAPTER 17

But Whats Your Real Name

It was February when I met my beautiful bride while back in Red Deer, the town we both lived in. I was back to get my gear in order and wait for the next call for work. While I was driving around I noticed I needed a new wiper blade for my truck, so I headed off to Superstore to buy one. This is where it all happened, kids. Here is where I met your mom for the first time.

I picked out the blade I wanted and headed toward the till. The grocery store was kind of dead at whatever time I was there, and the cashier (who would be my future wife) was waiting for a customer to scan their purchases. Well, she wasn't exactly just standing there. She was doing the pee dance—you know, the one where you have to pee so badly you slightly cross your legs and bounce up and down? She had a break coming up in a couple minutes and had convinced herself to wait instead of asking for a pee break.

Anyway, it was so freaking adorable, I just had to go to her checkout and investigate more. I think I said something like, "Do you have to pee?" And of course she said no, but then she continued the conversation to say how she liked my eyes. Hmmm. *You've got this, Kom-Tong, now seal the deal,* I thought to myself. So I said, "What's your name?"

She looked down at her name tag and said, "Ummm, Bambi," like I was some moron who didn't know how to read. So I said what everyone asks her when she tells them her name for the first time: "But what's your *real* name?" She of course said, "Bambi." So now I felt pretty stupid and really needed to put on the charm. Now came the best part, the time when I sealed the deal. I said ... "OK, bye."

That's right, kids, your father chickened out!

But as I was walking out, I thought, *You stupid moron, did you really just do that?!?!?! Man, I suck.* So I hopped into my truck and drove off. But don't worry, kids, I'm not done with this story yet. This frog does get the princess as you know because If I didn't, you two wouldn't have been born.

I was feeling like a total failure, as I knew I had missed that opportunity. But I thought there was still a way I could salvage this, and, as I have now taught own my kids, that Kom-Tongs never give up, even if it feels like you have failed. I thought to myself there has to be a way I can salvage this , so I came up with this not-so-ingenious plan. You may think it's stupid, but hey, I got the girl, so it wasn't *that* stupid!

About four or five hours after I got my wiper blade, I worked up the courage to call the grocery store and ask if Bambi was there. Of course, her shift had ended, but was I willing to try again the next day? Nope! I wanted to get that girl *now*! Trust me, when you see a girl like this, it's a once-in-a-lifetime thing. And if you don't act on it, you will miss your opportunity. So I told the woman on the phone that I was a new employee at Subway (which was connected to the grocery store at the time) and that I was talking to Bambi and she'd said she would give me a ride to work in the morning. I said I had forgotten to get her number and I needed it to make arrangements. Of course, they wouldn't give some stranger her number, which I figured would happen, so I gave them my pager number and asked them to pass it on to Bambi. Bambi was at Tony Roma's celebrating her birthday dinner with her parents when she received the call from her work.

Here was her side of the story: Her cell phone started to ring, and she saw that it was her work. She debated whether to pick it up. She had already worked a double and didn't want any more extra shifts. But she took pride in her job too, so she chose to answer the phone. She said right away, "Please, guys, I already told you I can't cover any more. I'm drained." Then they of course said it wasn't about that, that some guy named Jason had called and left his pager number because she was to be giving him a ride to Subway the next day. She thought to herself, *Ummm I don't even have a car,* but she took the number anyway, out of curiosity and said nothing else. She paged me, and I called her right back.

Normally that would be a fun story about how we met all on its own, but there is far more to it, because your father is not as smooth a guy as he thought he was.

When I called her, I invited her out for supper that night for all-you-can-eat ribs at Tony Roma's, and she told me she is already there with her parents. Well, that kind of blew up in my face. Then I asked her if I could pick her up later that evening and take her out for dessert, and she said YES!!!! So awesome. I had a date with the prettiest maiden in all the land. Kids, I know you don't want to hear this, but your mom is HOT. Like, super sexy hot!! So I was stoked. I had a date with this gorgeous girl after I had the all-you-can-eat rib fest at Tony Roma's with my friends. It was going to be such a great evening.

With some newly built-up confidence, I happily went to the restaurant and we ate like kings!! Rib sauce was flowing from my chin as I bore down on the next slab of bone and meat. Never before had I eaten myself into a food coma, but that's exactly what I did that night. I ate so much, I swear it was going to rip out from my skin. After dinner, I drove my friends home, knowing I had this date coming up with this beautiful girl. I dropped them off and had about thirty minutes to kill before going to pick up Bambi. I wanted to be punctual so that I didn't disappoint, but because I'd eaten so much, I decided to lie down in my truck (while it was still running) and take a quick power nap before my date because I was so, so full. Well, my quick power nap turned into a full night's rest. I woke up hours later, freezing cold because I had run out of fuel in my truck and had totally missed my date, all without knowing she had excitedly cancelled some of her birthday celebration so she could be with me. As far as I was concerned, I had slept through my only opportunity to impress and, at this point, it wasn't ever going to happen because I'd effed the whole thing up. So I gave up. (But, kids, it was a darn good thing your mom didn't.)

A few days went by and Bambi was chatting with her roommate about why the hell I hadn't shown up. It was really bothering her, more for closure than anything. What changed to make me not show up and was it something she said. She was clearly upset over thins and her roommate said, "It's the twentieth century and you didn't do anything wrong so call him and find out what the hell." So she did.

When I got the page, I was in the mall talking to my buddy about getting some Chinese food. I was interrupted by this buzzing in my pocket and was delighted and shocked to see her number pop up. So without hesitation, I rushed to call her back, not knowing how this was going to turn out. I wanted so badly to explain what had happened, but I was also so embarrassed. When I called, guess what she said to me. She said, "I'm not sure what happened the other night, but do you want to come over to my place and hang out? We are ordering in some Chinese food!" WHAT, ARE YOU SERIOUS????? *Throughout my life, you have always been just a step ahead of me. You were at the restaurant where I wanted to go, and you already ordered the food I wanted, before I even knew I wanted it.* There was something special happening here.

I headed over to her house, and the rest is history!!!!! We obviously hit it off, and this solo team became a team of two!

CHAPTER 18

The Great Promotion

Do you remember when you were young and you were always asked, "What do you want to be when you grow up?" Most of us replied: policeman, fireman, garbage truck rider guy! Really, if you think about it, we prepare our kids to be workers right from day one: What do you want to do? How are your grades? What college are you going to? What are you studying? And the last question you will be asked on a regular basis when you are all grown up: What do you do for work?

It's funny how we are all taught that having a job is the most important thing in life. Life should be about the memories you make and how you want to be remembered, or how you want to make a change/name for yourself in this world—not what you do to earn a living

We focus so much on work that we don't really focus on what's happening in front of us. Even when I was home, I had my mind so engulfed in my work phone or company computer that I didn't really know what was happening around me, and I definitely wasn't thinking how I looked in my kids' eyes. They would ask me a question or want to play and, because I was so focused on work, I barely, if at all, acknowledged their existence. Now I couldn't even imagine seeing this through the eyes of a kid, when the parents are so engrossed in their phone that they don't even take their eyes off to look at their kids while talking to them. I didn't realize I was working so much that I was missing out on so many memories I could have had with my family.

While I was in that hospital bed wasting away, I thought back on memories with the family, and all I could remember were the big things, like buying our first house or truck. I didn't have any memories of helping the kids with schoolwork or watching them play in the back yard. Now, because I have been forced to "retire from my job," I realize how much I missed out on because of work. I really wish I had found a good balance, but what I found important back then really wasn't important at all. Any kid would give up the nicer house or extra toys just to get the attention they deserve and desire from their parents.

I can't really speak for women, as I am not one, but speaking for men in general, we typically show love in the form of financial stability, by continuously working. But I figured out that isn't what matters. What matters is taking the time to talk to your partner and letting them know you are there to support them and take on interests and hobbies. Its all about finding that right balance and I didn't learn that lesson until after I got cancer. As I mentioned earlier, I came from a high school that was very technical with computers, as well as business orientated; they frowned on anyone who wanted to work a blue-collar job. When I was in high school, I saw myself as a mechanic in the military, so when I said I just wanted to be fixing things, the teachers basically wrote me off.

I did apprentice as a mechanic for some time during my high school years, but the oilfield was where I decided to go after graduation. I worked my way up, but how I got my management promotion was really a joke. My employer had no idea that I took night courses in the summer during my senior years in high school in small business management, or that I had been the manager for our school's football, basketball, and rugby teams. Honestly, I just had a knack for management but didn't ever embrace that—not yet, anyway.

To me, all those kids I went to school with worked their asses off to get the best grades and go to university, just to get a massive student loan and face huge amounts of competition when they entered the workforce. Everyone did the same thing (like sheep), and they all went into computers and business. Meanwhile, I had no student loan and constant work and beat people out for the position they trained so hard for, because I worked hard and got the real-life experience, not just the book version of how business works!

My life-changing career opportunity came when the manager quit in an act of rage. With the way our company operated, without the manger there even for a day, everything fell apart. Remember, we all have a structure we must follow or else there would be mass confusion and things would shut down. Well, it happened, and no one knew what to do, myself included. Then after about twenty seconds of utter silence, the phone rang. Not really knowing anyone in the office, I stepped up to answer it. I talked to the person on the other end about where the next job would be and took down all the numbers and lined up the job. I looked up and saw the owner standing at the office door. "Do you have this handled?" he asked.

"Well," I said, thinking it wasn't hard to take down directions and line up equipment for a job. The next thing I heard, out of the blue, was, "Well, OK, you are the manger now!" And he walked out of the building and drove back to Calgary. Seriously, that's how I got moved from a field worker into a corporate representative of our company. I was the company rep, the new manager. Nothing to do with the small business management certificate I worked so hard for over the summer while my friends were partying and planning trips. Not because I always busted my ass to ensure the jobs always went perfectly and without a hitch, but because I picked up the phone and wrote down some directions ... lol. Sometimes you still need to luck out regardless of how hard you work for it, but getting the opportunity and keeping it are two totally different things, I dominated that job because I trained for it.

The next time I saw the owner was about three weeks later. He was a tricky son of a bitch, he walked up to me, threw his hand out to shake mine, and announced that my salary was $60,000 per year at the same time we started the shake. ! Wait, what? No negotiation? We were already shaking, so I just accepted it. It wasn't nearly what I thought a manager would make, but I knew regardless where I started from , I knew there was no limit to the amount I could get to

So that was that. He was so quick on the draw, and if I shake on something, that's it, no ifs, ands, or buts. Even though this promotion was a great opportunity, I had to say it was not expected and it did make things a lot harder on my relationship. Still, I knew it was best to continue with it, as it was an opportunity that wouldn't come around again anytime soon. It was a life-altering jump into the office from the field, and I had no choice but to take it, regardless of how it messed up my personal life. Running a million dollar business that operates 24 hour a day, 7 days a week, ment that I was on call and expected to work whenever needed, and for a lot less pay than I was making in the field.

We were planning on having kids and had agreed that if we did, she would have a real career in case I was ever hurt or killed at work. I wasn't a manager when we had this conversation as this happened years earlier when kids were first brought up. . We made our plans for the future based on the nature of my job and the chances it presented for being injured while on the job. Having her pursue a career before children was the smartest choice we have ever made. This was a key factor in our financial survival as parents, as well as in how we pulled through the cancer stages of my life.

We figured the best bet for us to get ahead was to have Bambi move to North Vancouver with my mom and go to school to become a dental assistant as I worked as a well-testing day supervisor a couple months at a time before flying back to her on my scheduled days off, typically one week a month.

But that's how life goes sometimes. I had to jump at the manager position in Alberta with the pay decrease and sleep in my best friend's storage closet so I didn't miss out or screw up on this opportunity. (I *literally* slept in his storage closet ... yeah, we were living the high life back then!) Not so much, but this is what we needed to do to make it. Sadly, with becoming a manager, I worked in the office five days a week and had only two days off where I still needed to be close by in case something went wrong, so Bambi and I didn't see each other much while she was in school. We were in separate provinces, over a twelve-hour drive away.

Not seeing each other for six months at a time was something we had to sacrifice to get where we needed to be. We never intended to be apart that long, because when we planned it and registered her into dental assisting school, I should have been back one week a month as a field worker.

CHAPTER 19

Proposing to My Wife and to Work

During the time Bambi was in school, she came up to Red Deer to come to my Christmas work party. While getting ready for the party at her parents' house, I dropped to my knee and proposed to her in front of the Christmas tree. It was perfect because I'd planned for her mom to already be taking pictures of us looking amazing, so I was able to capture that moment in time. Bambi almost collapsed when I dropped to my knee to ask if she would become my wife. Without hesitation, she said YES! Then off we rushed to my work Christmas party, feeling pretty excited! The day I proposed to my wife, she got to witness what a great supporter I would be and my position within the company. I was the second highest ranking corporate rep at the party, and she got to see me in all my glory. And I got to show off my soon-to-be-bride to my employees. As far as life was going, we had it all! She was on track with her new career, we were going to seriously start working toward a future and family, and I was successful in my career. The next step? To plan a wedding!

The next time I was in Vancouver to see my fiancée, which was just around the Christmas holiday, there was a bridal show going on. I am not the kind of person who likes that kind of stuff, but Bambi was into it because I had just recently asked her to be my wife. So, knowing the idea was totally foreign and fresh in her mind, I decided to give in to her request, and with a couple of friends, we took off for the show. I have never been witness to anything like a bridal show. Brides-to-be are a different breed, demanding and loud—man, talk about crazy!!! It is the most important day of their lives, I am told, so I get that they want things their way and done to perfection. Personally, weddings aren't my thing. I would have liked a simple camping trip to celebrate and called it good. But we definitely didn't have that, because Bambi won the whole freaking grand prize wedding package!!!!!!

It was $35,000 in services you could use toward your wedding. So basically, with all these coupons for free or massively discounted services, she could get the wedding of her dreams. Talk about fate pairing us up, hey? Each venue at the wedding fair gave away something for free, or at a very discounted price—some things we didn't use because it wasn't smart. For example, there was a dress place that gave away $3,000 toward a new dress, though the cheapest dress there was $6,000. So technically it wasn't like we used the whole $35,000 and that it was fully covered, but it sure helped, especially with the photographer, DJ, and honeymoon to CUBA!!!! Those were all included/free and were a huge contributing factor to our perfect wedding, which was princess perfect, except for the heat.

The heat wasn't something we took into consideration when choosing our wedding day, and it was bloody hot out! The best thing that wedding package did for us was force us to have the wedding in Vancouver, because that's where all the services were based out of, so we didn't even have to discuss or fight over where we were having the wedding. Would it be in Red Deer, where she grew up, or Vancouver, where I grew up? In fact, the only thing we did fight about was the fucking tablecloths. One day, the stress just got to both of us, and the epic tablecloth fight was on! To this day, the word tablecloth is forbidden around our house. Seriously, you want to see fire protrude from her eyes, just say the word "tablecloth."

Our wedding was perfect for us, and when it was over, we headed off to the all inclusive resort in Cuba. Just before we took off, I left my job, as it was a whole new adventure, and I wanted a fresh go at it. I decided to break out internationally as a well-testing day supervisor. We talked about it before our wedding and decided this was the best career move for us at the time. I could earn a bunch more working internationally, and she would work as a dental assistant, learning the ropes of working in a dental office. We both were focusing on building a solid foundation prior to bringing kids into the world.

When we returned from our honeymoon, I started a new job with a friend I'd met years earlier who we will call Mr. Smith. During the time I was just starting the climb up the corporate ladder. I will always remember something he said when I started working with him. It became a key factor in my work ethic and how I present myself to this day. When I said to him, "Fine, if the office wants to play games with me, then I will play too," he said, "It's only a game if you want to play. You picked this job, so do the job, and if you want to complain about it, then just leave. You are in no way stuck here. We don't have anyone here who doesn't want to be here. If you don't like it, there's the door, because we don't need you. But if you face the problem like a man and figure out the solution to it, then please stay with us." After that, we became great friends!

Mr. Smith is an ex-military PPCLI sniper, and the story of his life just fascinates me. He had experiences I could only dream of, being a person who only ever wanted to join the military. The knowledge he has and the things he's experienced would just blow you away. And not just in his military life. I learned a lot from the stories of his past.

While catching me up and teaching me about this company for whom I was now going to work, Mr. Smith kept mentioning our new boss, who I knew I had to get to know. The manager to me was irrelevant at the time because they were so easily replaceable—hell, I became a manager because I picked up a phone when it rang. We all already knew the managers were glorified phone jockeys, which is what I learned during the years of doing the job. But the head boss … that was the guy I wanted to meet. His name was Mr. Red.

So Mr. Smith showed me the phone list of all the new people I got to work with, and guess who one of them was. Guy. Fucking Guy, fuck me. Even to this day I think back to how he burned me on that helicopter job and how he disrespected me in front of my crew. I even thought about not taking the job for a second, but I knew the pros outweighed the cons and that it would be a matter of time before Guy did something stupid. I just needed to face the problem and work it out of the equation. Kids, you need to learn this lesson: in life, you will come across people with whom you just won't ever mesh. But don't let that cloud your vision from your path. And always treat your fellow workers with respect, because you never know when you will be working beside them again. Remember, you must respect the position, not necessarily the person.

CHAPTER 20

The Return of the Village Idiot

Because I had already signed a contract with the company and was excited to work with Mr. Smith again, I decided to stay on and deal with working with Guy. When I was hired, it took the office a while to land a contract they'd been working on, so in the meantime, we all had to wait it out while sitting on salary. This was perfect, because I was setting up our new house, which we moved straight into after the wedding.

Not too much longer after I was settled in, we got that call, and I had to go to Rock Springs, Wyoming, and help take over for a division that was struggling to keep a manager. The old manager didn't like how head office was treating the guys so decided to walk out. Every employee followed. Honestly, that's the kind of manager I hoped to be when I was doing that role—one that people are proud to call their boss because they know you truly care for them and their families.

After I got the call, I did what everyone did when they received such a call: packed up my gear and headed down to Rock Springs. And who did I get stuck carpooling with but, you guessed it, Douchebag Guy! That was nineteen hours of driving with a human I hated so bad. I noticed a book in the back seat of the truck and decided to start reading it to avoid conversation. The book was a very popular novel back then, but I only picked it up to avoid having to talk to Guy. To my surprise, the book was so good, I actually didn't mind the drive, because I had nineteen hours to invest in finishing this amazing novel.

We arrived in Rock Springs and right away got thrown into this whole new division, and we were told to figure out the issues and make it work. I have to say that the whole team did amazing. About three months went by and our division was doing great! All of the guys did an amazing job re-organizing things, and we made the whole place user-friendly. We had space to work now, and things were going smoothly. Of course, out of habit, I still answered the phones, and before you knew it, I was standing face to face with our boss, Mr. Red. He came up to me one day and said he was impressed with my work ethic. Now maybe he said that to everyone, I don't know, but what I do know is that he sure made me feel good about myself, and I was quite happy there. I felt respected where I worked and like my opinion mattered, even if he was just blowing smoke.

More time passed and we had you, Zack, our baby boy, in 2008, which was a magical moment. It was something I was so looking forward to. I was so excited for the moment when I got to hold my newborn, who would look up at me, and I would feel a connection, a father-son bond that would never be broken. You know that feeling when your child is born and you feel an instant connection and the meaning of real love, because this baby is the best of both of you put together? Well, that didn't happen with me. It was nothing like my vision. It was more like, OK, this thing poops and cries, great—is that it? How boring! You see, I hadn't been there for most of the pregnancy, so I didn't really get to create that connection. But that's kind of how it goes with this kind of job. Don't get me wrong—I was far from a deadbeat dad. I helped with it all: feedings, diapers, and puke, while doing house stuff because, from the C-section,

Bambi was still not that mobile. It just wasn't what I expected at all, it was just tasks.

About a month went by and I got the call to get back to work. About two weeks into the job, I was having a couple of drinks with the managers and my new boss, Mr. Red, when who walks into the pub? It's fucking Guy. And what does he do? He talks non-stop about how great a job he did when I worked for him and how he moulded me into what I am today. If he meant how I hate disrespectful little liars, he would be correct. But he didn't mean that at all. He meant it in a way that, if it wasn't for him, I would have been lost and wouldn't have known what to do.

Then he went on to tell them how they'd offered him a battery operator job where he had to travel by helicopter and they would provide a cabin for him to stay in, and then he went on about how he turned it down, as it wasn't what he wanted to do. I CALL BULLSHIT! By this point, I was really pissed off because of his lies, so I decided to encourage him to have more drinks to see what would happen next.

After supper, the managers and boss left, but I decided to stay behind to talk with Guy. We started talking about what he wanted out of life, and he started bragging about how bad-ass he was and that he was planning to get a tattoo of all the deadliest snakes in the world on his neck. Two more hours went by and we were having a pretty intense conversation, but somehow I convinced him that a corn snake (which is actually harmless) was the deadliest snake in the world, so he insisted he get it tattooed on his neck that instant. So I paid for our drinks and we headed out for a walk. And, lo and behold, we came across a tattoo shop just down the block.

We walked in and the most incredible thing was happening right in front of my eyes. A white supremacist supporter was demanding that the artist put a swastika on his neck, and the artist was refusing to do so. The artist stuck to his morals and refused to be a part of problem that spreads fear in others, so the tattoo artist ended up escorting the guy out. He did it in a really respectful way. He even gave the names of some tattoo artists that would do it for him, he just said he didn't support that kind of art and what it represents. This kind of gave me a new view of tattoo artists. This artist diffused what could have turned into a bad situation by still holding on to his moral compass but giving him a way out. I turned to Guy and said, "Is this something you really want to do?" feeling a little bad about my part in his decision. But he said that he was going to do it, with or without me. I guess his mind was made up!

At the time, even though I now have a couple of tattoos, I found tattoos kind of thuggish, and not so much a thing of beauty. My wife got a tattoo later in life, and I consider it really classy. Her tattoo is a rendering of the speech wavelengths of all of us saying I love you to her. She interconnected the wave lengths of our voices in a coloration of colour and has that tattooed on her arm. Now *that* is beautiful!

Getting back to the story, because that guy got kicked out, we had a perfect window to get this "deadly" corn snake tattooed on his neck! Because a spot opened up. HAHAHAHAHA. Guy took his appointment slot. I figured this would be the perfect way to let people know the kind of person they would be dealing with. Really, it was his idea to put this warning sign on his neck, fully visible to everyone he met but I cant feel somewhat responsible. Even fifteen years later, we still think twice when we see someone with tattoos on the neck and face. This was just a warning sign to others to keep their guard up with him.

All I did was encourage his decision, and not only did he get a freaking corn snake tattooed on his neck, but this artist was absolutely terrible. He must have been a week into the job or less, which I couldn't have planned better if I tried. I wish I had a picture to show you, but it was the worst thing I had ever seen. You know how a dream catcher looks— the string is in a circle but only in straight lines, so every turn is an actual corner and not a smooth curve? Well, yeah, that happened here. It looked like a three-dimensional red-and-black stop sign with a small snake face poking out of the side of it. I laughed for days and days; I couldn't help myself. He had a picture of the least deadly snake all curled up in attack mode looking like it was made with Lego blocks. Hey, in my defense, it was his idea. I just gently encouraged him to follow through with his dreams.

A few weeks passed and Guy came to tell me he was going to buy a motorcycle, but he couldn't buy the specific bike he wanted in the US because they only let a certain number of those bikes into each country and him being Canadian they wouldn't seel it to him regardless where he was going to get it registered. I don't know if that's true, but either way, he was upset because he couldn't buy one. I felt a little bad for him and decided to help him with it. I figured out a way he could maneuver through a small loophole in the system, which really wasn't that hard. He just needed to figure how the motor vehicle system worked in the States and Canada and find the small differences where some paperwork might slip by, and it was all above board! He listened to my idea and followed my instructions and bought that Night Hawk or Night Rider, or something with the word "night" in it.

It was a really nice bike—it just had a goof riding it. I was glad to be able to help him a bit, because I did feel slightly guilty—not for the horribly drawn tattoo he had on the side of his neck, but that I had convinced him that the corn snake was a super bad-ass snake because it was able to survive so long without getting killed ... but still, so gullible!

It took a bit of time to get the paperwork handled, but when it went through, Guy was able to take his bike out for the first time. He rode it so proudly to the shop and, to be honest, the look worked for him. He had that whole biker vibe to him—not the tough, strong look, but the rough, weathered look. The kind a guy gets when he's lived a rough life.

He did the typical bragging thing, which all people should do when they get to buy their first bike, regardless of whether they're a prick or not, and then he took off to the bar. The next day I heard a story about his new bike and why it had scratches all over it—not like road rash scratches, but a dent and markings. It sure didn't look as good as the day before, and you could tell something was wrong. What happened, apparently, was that he'd driven up to the local biker bar and parked his bike and gone in for a few drinks. Not too long passed by and I guess some guy walked in and yelled, "Who owns that new bike out front?"

Guy stood up and said, "That's my fucking bike. What of it?"

Then the guy said, "You might want to pick it up off the asphalt!" I guess the asphalt had been so hot that day that when he put the kickstand down, it slowly sank into the pavement, and with the weight of the bike on just that small, thin kickstand in the heat of the summer ... well, the bike didn't have a chance and eventually fell over. Oh Guy, life really doesn't like you!

Not too much more time passed before Guy was arrested and extradited to Texas and thrown into jail—something about biting off some girl's fingers when he was super high. Seriously, I don't make this shit up!

Either way, he is now fully out of the picture, which makes me happy.

CHAPTER 21

My New Best Friend

Not long after that, I got a phone call from my beautiful wife to say she was pregnant with our second baby! GREAT!! I was super excited!!! I knew this time I would be more present for her pregnancy, because even though the last time we had done everything by the book to ensure a healthy, intelligent baby, I wanted to create that bond/connection with this baby prior to it entering the world.

With Zack, even though I did everything I needed to do for my baby in the beginning and onward—like change diapers and midnight feedings and such—I never saw the joy in it. Well, not until one day that I will never forget. It was just a typical day. My son was crying in the back seat for no real reason in one of those rear-facing seats. In fact, he was bawling, and while I want to say it was a cute cry, it wasn't. It just agitated the hell out of me hearing that damn noise. It was a shrill sound that pierced your ear, almost like a jagged piece of glass getting poked in your ear canal. It was like twisting metal, and I was just annoyed with it, right up until I put my one hand back next to him and the noise instantly stopped as his little baby hand grabbed three quarters around my finger and, all of a sudden, we were both at peace. Though he couldn't see me, he realized I was still with him and he wasn't alone, and he felt safe that I was there for him. And from that moment on, I was his daddy and not just "the boy's father." I would always and will always protect him. My heart melted for the little guy, and he became my best friend instantly. Sadly, it took that long to have that moment with my baby boy, but I was just happy it finally happened! Since then, I've done things out of love, not necessity.

So when Bambi called and said our second kid was coming, I was super excited! My daughter Kisenya came into this world with glowing blonde hair and majestic, crystal-blue eyes. I know lots of babies start with blue eyes and blonde hair, like my son, but after time it goes away, but for her it didnt. I look at myself with what used to be jet black hair, but these days it has more of a silver glimmer to it, and my shit-colored brown eyes, and I wonder how my beautiful brunette wife with hazel eyes and I ended up with a blonde, blue-eyed little girl.

Then I was reminded of our wedding day when my best friend who was also my best man, has blond hair and blue eyes . And I recalled how during my wedding he leaned over to kiss my wife. Hmmm, made a guy think. But I knew that couldn't be it. Why that actually happened was that he was sitting up at the wedding party's table having his supper two seats away from my wife while I was across the banquet hall getting a refill on my beer and talking with my good friend, Bart, who was our bartender. All of a sudden, someone started clinking their glasses as they seem to do at all wedding receptions. Well, I was far across the banquet hall and nowhere to be found, so what did my best man do? He stepped up to the plate, leaned her back in her chair, and gave her a kiss on stage with all my family and friends watching. I'm not sure that's actually in the rule book for a best man, but thanks for stepping up, bro … I think? Because of that, we always joke that he might be the father. But we all know he's not.

Though the window was a small one, because I was usually away at work, make no mistake, Kisenya, that you are 100% a Kom-Tong! Bambi tries to explain to me that it has to do with Y chromosomes and Z vitamins, and Q hormones … yeah, I still *don't* get it, but according to her, some dominant gene can come into play and change people to blonde or blue eyed or even albino. So sweet heart, if you ever wonder why you are blond and blue eyed, just ask your uncle Steve!

Kids, I assume you will find this the most interesting part of my story because this part is the part that really tells the story of the birth of our family. Before I continue, I want to share a couple of funny stories about your names. Zack, when you were born, we were sure you were going to be a girl and had a girl's name picked out, Kadence. But in the unlikely possibility you were a boy, we were going to call you Zackary or Lincoln. I was so positive you would be a girl, I didn't really fight for the boy names but if I did think you were going to be a boy, I would have fought more for Steel or Doctor. Mom was leaning more toward Lincoln, and I liked both but was leaning more toward Zackary. Your mother wanted nothing to do with the names Doctor or Steel. I liked those names because, believe it or not, there is power in a name. If we went with Doctor, no matter what you decided to do in life, people would have to call you Doctor, which would automatically earn you respect when meeting someone for the first time, especially when you were older. And Steel would have made anyone subconsciously think of you as one tough son of a gun!

If you had to pick a strong, powerful person just by their first name, who would you pick? A Eugene or a Brad? Sorry to say, but as you can see from my stupid little experiment, I am right. So no matter what, I was going to make sure your name had some power to it. But regardless the power in the first name, you are a Kom-Tong, and we are tough as nails! But your mom was standing her ground with a firm NO to Steel and Doctor, and thinking you were most likely a girl, we didn't 100% decide on a name. But, seriously, if you *were* named Doctor, how awesome would that be? Everyone would call you Doctor Kom-Tong, and you wouldn't have even had to go to school. You would get that title and I wouldn't have had to pay your university. Thanks a lot, hon. Now Zack will have to get an education. How lame!

But here is a funny story how I got to pick your name behind your mom's back. Mom had just finished delivering you and was still groggy from the C-section medicine, so when the nurse handed me the forms to register your name, I looked over at Mom to make sure she was completely out of it. I grabbed something to write with and wrote in that your name would be Zackary William Kom-Tong, as I liked it a bit better than Lincoln. Your mom's choice was always Lincoln, which she confirmed when she woke up. When she looked over at the form she said, "What the hell? Did you fill out his name?"

"I did," I said.

"That's not the name I wanted," she said.

"It's OK, honey, we can change it if you like," I said but then added, "but I think it's written in pen." Sorry, not sorry! And that's why you are called Zackary William Kom-Tong!

As for your name, Kisenya, what a difficult task that was. Ugh, I could have killed your mother for the agony she put me through trying to come up with your name. If you were boy, we knew what it was going to be, of course!!! DOCTOR!!!!! Just kidding. It would have been Lincoln. Funny side story here: when I was filling out your name on the sheet, I saw a new section that said I was not allowed to use the name "Doctor." Maybe that section wasn't new, but I don't recall seeing that on Zack's form. Maybe when Zack was born and I told our nurse I wanted his name to be Doctor she ripped me a new one for disrespecting her profession. Maybe it pissed her off enough to do something about it. Who knows?

Kisenya, if you were a girl, we had no clue what to call you, and your mother would not stop freaking nagging me to pick a name that we both loved. Kadence was not allowed to be an option for some reason, probably because she was bitter that the name she'd wanted was axed, so it's quite possible she wasn't letting me have that just to spite me. Or maybe because Kadence was turning into a more common name. Either way, all I ever heard from her was: "What about this name? What about that name?" over and over and over and over and over. You seriously don't understand how annoying it was. Every person we met, or show we watched on TV, or things we passed by while driving: "What about fire hydrant, grass, or autumn rain?" After literally hours and hours each day, I was just agreeing to any name to shut her up so I could quietly watch a football game or have a full conversation without being interrupted.

Then one day your mom ended up saying a name she thought she'd heard a woman call her daughter that had caught her ear, but she didn't have a full grasp of it. She was close but couldn't get it exactly, so Bambi walked up to her and said, "What was that name? It was so pretty." And the woman said it again, and it wasn't even close to what she'd heard. Still, Bambi thought she'd heard a name that just sang to her, so when she came home, she asked me in a more serious way with this look in her eye: "What do you think about the name Kisenya," which I without a doubt immediately also loved. We both knew from that second forward that if we had a girl, we were calling her Kisenya! I like to think one of the signs of love for your baby is not only the fact that you created such a beautiful thing through the love and bond you share with the other parent— and both my lovely babies are the most beautiful babies in the world to us—but giving our daughter her own identity, knowing she is the first Kisenya in this world! At least that we know of. Daddy loves you princess and you too Zackary (AKA Steel) !!!

I must say, I couldn't have asked for two better kids. They make me laugh when I need it, they pick me up when I am down, and they make me feel like I am always someone who's wanted and needed. They've both stepped up to the plate when I've needed them the most.

Because of my diagnosis and surgeries, Zack had to learn to read at a way younger age than normal, and on a way higher level than normal, just to communicate with me. The two of them had to learn at a very young age that their dad was going to leave forever and very soon, and even though it wasn't their fault and there was nothing they could do, they were going to be left without a daddy.

This was my sole reason for never giving in to suicide. As long as I was able to keep going to the end of the day, or the next morning to say good morning, then I damn well was going to be there to see them one more day. Plus, they gave me lots to do.

CHAPTER 22

From Alaska To Africa

After we had Kisenya and prior to getting cancer, things were looking good in my life, and I was happy. And then I got told I would be heading to Alaska to work on a long-term contract. So, like many times before, I packed my things and got on the plane.

My first flight transfer was in Juneau, which is an amazing place to see. But I didn't stop there long enough to really look around before being sent to the northern slope. Brrrrr and brrrrrr. And talk about isolation. The camp was amazing, but once you were there, that was it. You were literally there and only there! Nothing but flat. Miles and miles of flat, blinding-white surroundings. You were quite literally forced into utter isolation.

When I first walked into the camp, it was really nice and well kept. I thought, *Wow, these guys are spoiled.* There was a gym and a movie theatre, and the food was great every night. But like I said, you were isolated much like we all were when covid-19 impacted the world. But until with what happened with covid, as per my employment agreement, my contract stated that I worked three weeks on and one week off so being isolated from the world wasn't too bad because I knew I would see my wife and kids soon enough. That was my schedule—or so I was told.

Up in the camp there was also this woman who looked like a wrinkled-up old witch with a teardrop tattoo under her left eye. We talked a few times in passing, and every time I saw her, I thought she must have been about eighty. If she was any younger than that, then life must haven't had been very kind to her… if you catch my drift. Either way, for the most part I kept my distance from good old tear drop because she really creeped me out. But sixteen days into that kind of isolation, where you can't really go outside for any period of time except for work, I found myself chatting her up like from the star football player in high school would have done to the newest pretty girl that transferred from Sweden. I was acting all cocky and leaning up against the wall—you know in that way where you're kind of blocking her path, acting all cool and slick. And I was like, "So what are you up to tonight, tear drop?"

At that point, I realized that I had to get the hell out of there!

I decided to check into my departure date for home, which meant looking up emails, which was only doable with the camp computers that were set up along the front entrance hall. There were five desktop computers in a row across the wall in the coat area, which was a massive space for all the coverall coats, bibs, boots, and other winter gear.

I had to check it quickly because I was about to head out to run the night shift, not that it mattered, because in the winter, it was always a night shift on the Northern Slope. Not seeing any return flights home or emails, I sent an email to the Alaska division asking if they would send me my flight information, as I had five days left and hadn't received any tickets yet. A couple more days went by and there was still no reply. I was getting a little frustrated, because I was on a twenty-ten schedule and I should have been preparing to head home by then, so I sent another email to the Alaska manager requesting it, and I made the drive off to my night shift. After work that morning when I got back, first thing I did was check my email.

And what did I see but an email from the manager's secretary stating that I would be up there for as long as they needed me, and that they would not be getting me a plane ticket until they were good and ready to send me one.

Well, here is a very important lesson I should have learned way earlier in life: DO NOT SEND AN EMAIL IN ANGER! YOU WILL REGRET IT. But I did just that. I sent an email off and just tore into them. I told them how unprofessional they were and how the secretary was a complete $%^&*, and how dare she talk to me like that, and how they can't manage shit, and I just ripped into them.

Normally if they said I was to work extra time that would have been fine, but you don't wait until the guy is in his five-day count-down, getting ready to go home and see his family. At that point, all I was thinking about was my family and how excited I was to see them, and this stupid job threw a wrench into any plans I had. I should never have sent that, and for that I am sorry. But I did send it, and that's how I was feeling at the time and I didn't give a shit, because "I hate you all and I just want to see my wife and kids, so FUCK YOU!" AND ... SEND!!!

Oh my gosh, what the hell had I just done??? Why did I send that? Oh shit, what was I going to tell my wife? Oh no, how could I face her and tell her I'd lost all our financial security and was jobless, and that we would probably become homeless? What had I done? How would I pay for our house? After sending that email, I thought, *I must be the stupidest person in the whole world.*

So off to the worksite I went, where we didn't have internet or even a cell connection. The drive to work was about ten minutes, and as soon as we arrived, the first thing the cross shift said to me was "Dude, what did you do? I can't believe you still have a job after that." Seriously ... what? I instantly felt like puking up my guts. I had to work for twelve hours, wondering why I'd sent that and was convinced I was fired, and more importantly, agonizing over how I would tell my wife and family. The good thing was that I was sure I was heading home, and maybe even earlier than the two more days on my contract. So after what felt like an eternity, the cross shift came in and of course wanted to know if I still had a job—and to be honest, I wondered the same. I packed all my gear into the company truck and headed back to camp to check my email.

I parked and slowly dragged my ass into the camp, hanging my head as low as a man can while still walking upright. I sluggishly made my way to the computer and, not to my surprise, there was a new unread email in my inbox from my boss, Mr. Red. It took me a second to realize it, but this email came to me as a CC. It wasn't actually directed to me. Huh? It was an email from my boss to the Alaska boss that said, "If Jason has a problem with you, then there's a damn good reason he's voicing his opinion. You better get off your lazy ass and get my guy home as per his contract, and that goes for all my guys. I will pull every fucking worker I have from your division. I am helping you out because you couldn't see a couple weeks into the future. And he better be home in two days as planned, and that's final!"

Ummmm … WTF had just happened?!? Had my boss just stuck up for me?? I had never seen this before. I didn't know what to say, but holy shit, had I ever dodged a bullet there, and I promised myself I would never do that again. To this day, I've sent out everything strategically and professionally, for the most part. I may try to joke around here and there and attempt to catch a person who doesn't have a sense of humor off guard, but that's just what I do to some people. But I never email in anger anymore. If I'm mad, I must wait until I can think rationally and weigh all options before I document something in writing that can be traced back to me.

That day, I learned I could trust Mr. Red not only as a boss but as a person who would look out for me and would support me in bettering myself. I don't regret that decision, not for a second! To this day if you ask him about this, he won't remember doing that at all, and that's because of the kind of guy he is. He will always stick up for the guy who has been wronged, and he will always respect his employees as people! You know, he never even brought this up, not even the day after that email. To him, it was nothing. But to me, it was everything. Thank you, Mr. Red, for always having my back when I needed you. You are a true friend and a nice, trustworthy guy!

More time passed and my job had me travelling not only throughout the US, but also off-shore in Scotland and Africa too. The Africa division wanted to keep me there, but to tell you the truth, after my first hand experience there, I will never go back. This scheduled stint , would be one that would scar me for life and would give me a whole different outlook on the world around us. Did I expect to see the scene set in my head by TV when they ask for donations for African communities that need medicine and fresh water, yes of course.....I know some may hear Africa and think the beautiful tundra with Lions and Zebras, But when you work the oilfield, you don't go to places that are ever visited by tourists, so I did expect the worst, but expecting it and living it are two totally different things. The place was actually quite magnificent if you could look past the poverty and the government structure. When I arrived I was instantly treated like royalty and it was only because I was from a First-World country, I was considered the boss when I arrived, and man did they ever roll out the carpet. So much so that I didn't even have to go through customs. There was a guy waiting for my arrival where he paid off the customs agent and I just walked in. My personal security guards took my luggage and we go into the armoured vehicle and was transported into building that I can only compare to something like a parliament building. There was full time staff, every luxury a person would want all within the walls of the compound. My team of employees who I had to boss around were guys who spoke four languages fluently and were engineers and more, and here I had to tell them to move this heavy pipe around, hammer it together, and go paint equipment. Consciously I knew it was wrong, as these guys were way smarter than me but had just been born into a harder life. I was privileged by my class structure, when in reality I should have been working for them. I knew it, and deep down I hope they knew it too, but most likely they didn't because all their lives and everything they were taught since birth, was to do as they were told by people that held a higher title than them , and just to take it. I am so glad I don't live there as I personally know it's a lot harder life to live. Imagine just knowing someone is doing something wrong or less effective, but never being allowed to speak up and say so. I tried to have my guys teach me new tricks or better more efficient ways to do things, but I could tell they never were given the freedoms to speak up before and were very nervous when I asked for their suggestions

Oh, and a side note: just because we are Canadian doesn't mean we all speak French. It would have been nice if my international company knew that! I was in Abidjan, a French-speaking city on the southern Atlantic coast of Côte d'Ivoire in West Africa, and I didn't know a damn word in French besides "le hamburger." Thank God for the fellow workers who were there and could help translate for me. They all knew how to speak English as well as French. If it wasn't for them, I would only have been able to eat "le hamburger" at every meal.

The language barrier made for a hard time when we went through a security check and they pulled me aside to drill me with questions. I remember this one incident where a guard grabbed my passport and screamed some French shit into my face and walked off with it. If I'd known French, I would have known that he wanted five dollars to get it back. Instead, I jumped out of the vehicle and ran through over a dozen military personnel to keep track of, and catch up to, the only guard who didn't have an assault rifle strapped to his shoulder. I was told that at no cost was I to lose my passport or else I would have major issues when it came to leaving the country, my work visa and daily security. It was seriously an intense situation. But I found the guy and I got my passport back—but not without some memorable confrontations.

I found out in a hurry that it is important to always be informed about the countries you are going to visit and about their culture and how to protect yourself and be safe. Had I done that, I may have been prepared for something that I witnessed in Africa that literally broke my heart and scarred me for a long time. Every day, we were transported in an armed vehicle, where I would have my own personal guard to protect me. Now, you may be asking yourself where my guard was when we hit that road check and I lost my passport. What happened with that was the manager wanted to take us out somewhere nice for dinner, and against my better judgment, I went with them off the compound without any of the guards. We took a cab, as it was not really allowed. We were supposed to stay in the work compound, so really it was my fault for being a sheep and putting myself in a bad position. I knew better but didn't want to be the odd man out.

But what I was about to experience was absolutely horrific, the opposite from my typical day-to-day trip to the dock when we were in between offshore jobs. There was one major streetlight that we always got stuck at, and every day we saw this little girl, probably about eight years old, standing at this same corner begging for money. When the light turned red, she would walk up to any car that had a white person in it and wave, praying they would give her money to feed her and her poor grandmother, who would be sitting in her wooden wheelchair on the side of the road—literally, a wooden wheelchair. The first couple of times I saw her I wanted to give her some money because I felt bad for her and her shriveled-up grandma, plus she reminded me of an older African version of my daughter: diligent, outgoing, and so damned innocent. But my guard would never let me give her anything. Almost every time we stopped at that light, I tried to reach for my wallet, but he would grab my wrist and shake his head no at me, so I eventually stopped trying. Then one day I was so happy because, as we slowed to a stop, I saw her get some money from the car in front of us, and she had the biggest smile on her face. Now, I have no idea how much she got, but it must have been good because she started to skip back to her granny, waving her hand with the money gripped in it so tightly. Then all of a sudden out of nowhere, a man came flying out of the bushes and, with all his might, smashed his fist into her face with his bare knuckles. The grandma screamed as the little girl's lifeless body was laid out cold on the ground. The man scrambled up all the fallen money and sprinted down the road. In a state of total shock and completely reactionary, I instinctively reached for my guard's assault rifle, and was ready and willing to kill this guy. It was so morally wrong in so many ways. This man needed to die, as far as I was concerned, and I didn't care what rules I was breaking. Seriously, what the fuck had just happened?

My guard, who had a grip on his gun so tight I could barely budge it, acted like nothing happened and said *that's just life* in Abidjan, and the motorcade proceeded as normal, making sure not to run over the little girl's motionless body. To this day, I still think about that girl and how that must have affected her, if she even survived that. It broke my damn heart. At this point, I had no idea how much time I had left there, but I knew that would be my last trip to Africa. That really fucked me up, and I struggled with trusting people for a long time.

CHAPTER 23

Back On Home Turf

But there was one man I did trust without question, and that was my boss.

When I got back home about one month after that incident, a few things changed. For one, I was contacted by Mr. Red, who told me he had been let go during the months I was in Africa and had found a well-testing company based out of Red Deer where he wanted me to work for him as one of his operations managers. So with Mr. Red's full trust in me, I was able to start up a division for that Red Deer-based company in North Dakota! The other manager who had been brought on was having some issues crossing the border from Canada due to an old drinking and driving record he had gotten years before in the States. So with the direction of Mr. Red, I was able to set up the whole company, from the ground up, as the only man with boots on the ground, so to speak! To this date, it is one of my greatest corporate achievements. But it will slide to a solid second place once I finish what I am currently working on.

By that point, I felt as though Mr. Red was a bit of a father figure to me. Just because I worked away so much, he was always there with me when I needed any kind of advice—from work stuff, or how to approach a problem, even to parenting techniques. There were two major things I learned from him that changed my life as a parent.

The first was a choice he and his wife had had to make way back when they were at the beginning stages of building their family. You see, their kids were and are really smart, and they had the option to put them into a normal school or a school for advanced learners. He told me they went with the former, because why single someone out who is gifted and seclude them and shelter them from the people with whom they will come in contact day after day? Let them use their gifts to get ahead in life. It wasn't exactly like that, but something along those lines, and I never thought of it that way. I assumed if they excelled at something it would put them into a special class where they would be challenged every day, and it couldn't hurt them. If a kid is good at something, don't change anything. Let them thrive in that environment they are in and excel at what they are doing. So my kids are currently in a normal school and not one for gifted kids, though they're smarter than most. Ask my wife how she ensured our kids would be super intelligent. It has to do with dolphins….yes I said dolphins.

If I could have had it my way prior to his advice, I would have them in a private school—not that I think it's much different, but I never had that option as a kid, and I want my children to experience both and let them decide their path. I realized that as long as they were happy in their current environment, I was doing what was best for them—in my opinion, that is. I'm sure others may disagree with me.

The other and probably best advice Mr. Red gave me was to create an amazing bond with my kids. His advice on what a spouse should do when they work away from the family on schedules like ours was so simple yet so important. He suggested that I send my wife on a week-to-ten-day vacation with one of her girlfriends while I stayed home with the kids. If I had to, he said, just pay for both of them to go if cost was an issue for the friend. He suggested that my wife should pick the place and person she wanted to take with her and just go and have a nice break. He said, "Do this if you want to create an impactful bond with your kids. Not only does your wife get a well-needed vacation with her friend, but it might influence her decision in allowing you to buy that boat she hasn't let you buy, but most importantly, your kids learn they can fully rely on Dad to take care of them when Mom's away." I needed to show them that Dad was just as good a caregiver and loved them just as much as Mom did. I owe that amazing bond and trust I have with my two kids to Mr. Red's advice. I know they would be completely different kids than they are today if I hadn't listened to that advice. So, in kind, my advice to anyone reading this who has small children is this: show them that you can and do provide for them as someone they can trust. Kids don't consider finances as important as personal relationships, so ensure that you show them how much you love them and tell them stories and make sure that you aren't just there to provide financial support for the family.

Honestly, in my life, and in all of our lives, for the most part, things were going great in this stretch. The business kept growing, and I was on the road to success. We even decided to move from our first house in Sylvan Lake to our new house in Red Deer, and this house was freaking fantastic! It was our forever home, the last move and final house for my family. So I thought. It had three living rooms, six bedrooms, four bathrooms, and it was perfect.

I spent every day off, for six months straight, looking for this perfect house for us and I never found it. I started to hate looking. You see, my new schedule was twenty-one days on and one week off, but two of my days off were a twelve-hour drive to work and back, so I was home for just five days a month. And for six months straight, all we did in those five days was look at houses, every day, all day. To Bambi, it was only five days a month, but to me it was *all* the time I got to spend with my family per month. So on day two of my next twenty-one-day shift back at work, when my wife called me to say she found the right house, I said, "Just buy the fucking house," because I just didn't care anymore ... lol. Yes, that actually happened. I said, "Just buy it!" I didn't care to look at it or even know the area in town. She had done this searching long enough to know what we were both looking for, and when she got the go-ahead for the purchase, she didn't mess around. She got all the stuff done with me at work and we did all the paperwork over the internet and via fax, and in less than twenty-one days, we had our second home!

And I have to say that Bambi did the most amazing job ever. She found our forever home! It was absolutely perfect and needed nothing extra. We loved it! I literally came home to a new house, my dream home! Things were going as planned. Beautiful wife, check. Two perfect kids, check. Great home, check. Financial stability, check.

CHAPTER 24

Loose baggage

It was around this time, when things were going so well, that I felt the newly formed laceration on my tongue. Unbeknownst to me then, this was the first real sign I had tongue cancer. It was the worst pain I had ever endured. This laceration had a mind of its own and would get really painful at times. At other times, it would just be a continuing painful reminder that something was wrong. There would be days at a time I would go without eating because it hurt so much, but then it would die down and go away for a while, only to return a week later, and we would do this over and over again for years. I went and had it checked out, and multiple times the doctor said it was nothing and that it would just go away. Each time, I was given some T3s for the pain and told it should clear up—which it would, for a short while, but then it would just come back again. This went on for a very long time, during which I got a new job with another well-testing company doing the same thing as before, starting up a new division in North Dakota. The reason I had to start this all over again was because Mr. Red got fired from his job (our previous employer), and what I believe happened, though I don't know for sure, was this ...

When my boss was initially hired on (from our last employer), he told the core corporate shareholders that he would build the company up (as he did), and they promised him a bonus of a certain percentage of their profits. They doubted his capabilities despite what he told them he could do and never expected their company to grow as fast and as successful as it did. Well, when he started off the new division, it took less than a month to get the start-up costs and payroll in the black. He had the contacts and business plan all organized before presenting the board with his projections. He shaped it in a way that the company expanded so quickly it had to buy up another one just to keep up with demand. Because of this, I suspect his annual contractual bonuses got kind of high. They figured out the mass expansions and growth prediction over the next couple years and thought it would be cheaper to fire him and pay his early termination rather than his bonuses. Really, business ethics and loyalty seem to be lost in the oilfield.

At that point, they asked me if I was going to leave with him, because they knew I looked up to him as a role model. But I said no and that I was truly going to stick it out there, not out of disrespect to Mr. Red, but in fact, the opposite: to honour him. I would apply all he taught me about business and make my project thrive and succeed and show him that everything he taught me about business and life and making the right decisions was not for naught. I knew it was time for me to stay and prove I had learned enough and was able to break out on my own. I talked to Mr. Red about this and he agreed that, though he would miss me, it was the right move for my career. That's another reason I loved working with him—he always pushed me in the direction that was best for me, regardless of whether it was best for him. So with his blessing, it was time to be on my own. Mr. Red, you taught me so much I needed to learn about business, and I wanted to see that company progress from start to finish, as it was my baby.

But what happened next is an example of another lesson learned. Some people will fuck you over, and there is nothing you can do about it. For me, writing this book was what I needed to do to prove to the world how cowardly some people can be.

About six months before Mr. Red was fired, the other manager finally got his work visa for the US and was able to do the job I had been covering while he was unable to cross the border. A few more months passed and the other manager, while working for our company, was also helping Mr. Red under the radar. He was getting quotes and lining things up for him and doing the research he would need to set up another well-testing division for another company. Mr. Red was just asking if he could help with getting some start-up numbers and quotes, and didn't dare ask me, because he knew it would be a total conflict for me. He knew when I said I was all in, it meant I was all in—and by the book. As for the other manager, he was all about himself. And if he thought for a second that he could get something out of something, he would for sure be a part of it.

Well, I shit you not, this actually happened, so pay attention kids, as this is something you will always need to watch out for. It's what we in the industry like to call the backstabber! This is the person who acts like your friend but only uses you for political gain, like some kind of pawn. Here's how that guy (my so-called friend) stabbed me in the back.

When I came back from our well-deserved family camping trip, I was fired out of nowhere. I was so confused and stressed out, all because someone had used me as a scapegoat so they wouldn't get in trouble.

After Mr. Red was terminated from our company, he found another company to whom he wanted to pitch the idea of starting up a new division in Minot, North Dakota. In gathering the info for his pitch, Mr. Red, who is always 100% accurate with his quotes and promises, asked the other manager to help get some quotes for him, with the promise that Mr. Red would hire him on when the new company started up. To help get these quotes, he ran it all through our current company name so he would get the best prices. As we had a very good reputation throughout the community. He had everything quoted and bundled. When they met up, the manager handed him the physical quotes in paper form, and Mr. Red put them in his travel bag, which he placed on the trunk of his car while they talked. When they were done talking, Mr. Red drove off, forgetting about the bag on the back of his car. Someone found his travel bag on the road, and when going through it in search of ID to find its owner. They must of found one of his old business cards from his previous employer (my company) and mailed the bag to head office.

When our corporate office received his bag, they went through it and found the quotes in our company's name but dated after Mr. Red's termination date. This is also how the head office found out there was a traitor within the company. Because of my obvious respect for, and loyalty to, Mr. Red, they all assumed it was me. But they were all fucking mistaken! The extent of the internal investigation consisted of making one phone call to the other manager and asking about these quotes they'd found in Mr. Red's travel bag, and opposed to manning up and telling the truth, the only thing he could think to come up with was, "It's not mine," implying: *Who else could it possibly belong to?* All fingers pointed at me.

I came back from my vacation to the manager telling me how he had "accidently" thrown me under the bus, and how he was sorry, which he tried to rationalize by saying at least I knew about it. I was a little worried about what corporate would say, but I wasn't that concerned because I'd done an amazing job for them and proven my character. Hell, as far as I was concerned, to me and everyone I hired on, the opinion was that I built that whole division from scratch, and they knew I would never jeopardize my job or my team . But alas, the HR manager of the company had already made up his mind, and I guess they didn't even want to hear my side of the story. Kam (one of the corporate managers) called a meeting with me at head office, where they fired me on the spot. He didn't even give me a chance to tell him what happened, you know, the truth. Hey, Kam, maybe you want to learn how to *actually* investigate a situation, "you useless dumb shit," because you lost a loyal employee and instead you kept a snitch that quit your company a week later anyway. You didn't even want to talk to me, let alone do an actual investigation. Here is the lesson in this scenario: *always* know both sides of a story before making a decision that will affect someone's life. No one's life should ever be affected negatively by someone not knowing all the correct information at the time of making a life altering decision.

So after getting fired, I was unemployed for about three hours, and I joke that that was the most stressful time of my life. But to be honest, it was actually the most peaceful and humbling three hours I've ever had. It was like all the doors suddenly opened and I was able to walk through any one I picked. Of course, I contacted Mr. Red, explained the situation, and he hired me on the spot. Shortly after that, we got together and started creating a new division for our new company. About a week later, the other manager came and joined our team, and we built up what was to be, a very powerful company. Obviously, I didn't trust the other manager from what he did to me in the past, so I kept a close eye on everything he did. You see, I knew he hadn't intentionally throw me under the bus when he did but the fact was he still did it and couldn't be trusted. I was just an easy out for him because he didn't want to get fired and lose his family's income, so he gladly passed it onto me to get himself out of the situation he created. What a looser and total chicken shit!

Some advice: if you are ever going to fire someone and drag them through the mud, you better make damn sure your actions are fully justified. Because the worst thing you can do is fuck up a guy's life with a decision based off an assumption. Just think, their company wouldn't have gone bankrupt if they kept me on, because when they let me go, 90% of the team jumped ship once they found out where I went. The company and investors literally lost millions because of this decision, but I don't think they had even thought of that until just now when I slapped them across the face with this book that tells them the real story Though the names were changed in my life story for publishing purposes, I'm sure they know who they are, and Kam, I do expect a long-overdue apology to me and more importantly my family for your unprofessionalism and lack of judgement. I do hope the old board of trustees and investors reads this book and realize they made a huge error in their corporate restructuring

Luckily I landed back on my feet but it could have been so much worse for me and my family. But don't worry, It was only a matter of time until I was able to get back at the other manager for not only rubbing our Kom-Tong name in the mud but jeopardizing our family's financial stability. The truth is, he had no care for what was to happen to me and my family's stability, and was all about trying to cover his own ass. He was the one that cast the first stone.

CHAPTER 25

Always look at the bigger picture

During the time I was managing the new well-testing company which meant overseeing hundreds of employees. I always had this belief that you needed to speak up and be heard if you wanted to get something done. because if you don't, your voice or idea would never reach the right level that could do something to make a change or impact. . But in addition to that, the person on the receiving end must be willing to actually listen or be willing to make a change. If not, the whole structure of a business will collapse.

One day, a worker of mine (a helper to one of my supervisors) woke me in the middle of my well earned sleep. The day ended with me, resolving an issue where two employees with personal issues, were stuck to work together on a split shift of 12 hours a day with travel time of 1.5 hours each way for 30 days straight. It was a job in Northern Alberta that was over 4 hours away from any city or town. That job, like every job we do, was the middle of no-where, in a vessel that's very tight to work in. I knew I had to resolve their squabble before it became not only a personal problem, but also a work problem. Oilfield guys range from some of the smartest people I know to some of the most stupid people. But no matter how smart or dumb you are, you put two men together for 30 days at 15 hours a day, they better fucking respect each other or else it makes for a bunch of very long days and very very long conversations. With these two it was all about a girl they both just recently found out they were both dating. Believe it or not, this situation came up more often than not, because when these guys come back from a long haul, they let loose as they didn't have to spend any money for the months they have been gone for and all the single available women in town know this and use them to party with. It's a hard life on these guys , as your work life ends up becoming more your real life, as its almost impossible to even keep a friend ship let alone a relationship alive when you are gone for so long. So when it came to my employees emotions, that was number one on my daily agenda over anything else, which was on top of all the usual accounting, purchasing, Internal and external audits, reporting, computer program updates, and the influx of daily safety reports, and incident cards that come in 24 hours a day 7 days a week.

My crews work 24 hours a day and 7 days a week, so when I'm on shift (my 20 days on and 10 days off) I am also expected to be available at all hours of the day or night just in-case there is an Incident or accident. I too worked away from home, so I was not uncommon for me to work 17-20 hours a day. I know if you don't keep up with the daily demand as well as the unforeseen add-ons like my employees issues. Then things will just fall behind which can rapidly burry an individual and even more importantly an entire business or corporation. I had a guy that filled in for me during my 10 days off which meant I couldn't let things fall behind even if I wanted it to as I knew he was wanting to find any excuse to take my job. At the time I didn't know how important this call would actually be, but it would change the lives of so many people with neither of us even realizing it. This call came in at 3am which meant there must be a somewhat urgent as my guys usually only contact me during the office hours. When he called he was very emotional, and passionate about what he had to say. It was the kind of call you would get from your best friend after he had long surpassed his drinking limit. But in this case I knew he wasn't drunk as he was at work during this time and the well they were flowing back was one of many safety professionals on location as this particular well was unstable. He had called to explain how he deserved a raise and promotion. "Really ? I thought to myself, you woke me up to ask for a raise, and you didn't think this could wait until I was at the very least awake? . I initially and irrationally thought to myself, there is no way in hell that you will ever get a raise now. I knew I couldn't just hang up on him and deal with it in the morning, as it would have been totally disrespectful. Also, as a person of authority, you never disrespect the ones who look up to you. So I was on the phone for two full hours, from 3:00 a.m. to 5:00 a.m., all while getting yelled at about how he deserved a promotion and was being forced to do something he didn't want to. He yelled with passion, and cried with emotion which made me remember how years ago I called my manager also around 3am to yell about that idiot I worked for. During this call with my employee, I realised there had to be a bigger picture that I just wasn't seeing, as this didn't come out from nowhere. After the call and after many hours of having this on my mind, I figured out what the real issue was. You see I realized that 2 years ago when I hired him, I also hired many other people to prepare for our expansion, and hes voicing his opinion to me with this kind of emotion, there might be others like him thinking the same thing, but just too scared to say it. I realized that others were also ready for a promotion to advance their careers. But at the time, I knew I didn't have any positions available to move them into. I didn't want to lose the workers I had trained and learned to respect and befriend. But I also didn't want to hold them back from their potential. I felt a little trapped but like anything, you just need to find the real issue and solve that and things will fall into place. I wasn't just a guy just doing a job, but I was also a guy doing a job that could seriously impact people's lives. If I didn't at least give him a shot at what I knew he felt he deserved, he would end up quitting and I would have to find a new person that would make the sacrifices and life changes to fit a job like this, Plus why would I want a guy that I trained and devoted hours of my time to help form him as a person and kick ass employee leave me to better another company and not mine?

People will be loyal to you if you treat them with respect and at the very least out of respect, I needed to at least try to help him out. . Look at any great leader and you will see it's not just them but their team that makes them great, and I wasn't willing to lose anyone from my team, regardless of their position or the time of day, or night, that they called me. But with no current positions available to promote him or anyone into as all positions are filled, what was a guy to do? The lesson is to always think outside the box, no matter the situation. There is always a way to fix a problem, you just need to find it.

The way our company ran was that we had two set shifts at twelve hours per shift, and each shift consisted of one supervisor and one helper. So I had to come up with a plan that pleased everyone and made the company more money , because it was a lot easier to get my bosses to approve any kind of change if it meant they also made more of a profit. The employees needed more money and we needed to provide more options for advancement within the company. I needed to figure out a way to create more jobs and, most importantly, make sure my guys kept progressing within their careers. Rarely in life are there times when everyone can be satisfied in a situation with minimal risks, but this was one of those times. All it required was some extra thought and brainstorming to figure out how I could make this happen.

We had four people per crew to work each job. The main guy was a day supervisor, the middle guy was a night supervisor, and two assistants did most of the grunt work. After a lot of thought, I figured out the best way to please everyone. I figured out a way to give the day supervisor a twelve-hour shift that overlapped 2 other crews. Basically, I added a full position for each crew and an extra truck the company could charge for. I added one more experienced guy to each location and gave the day supervisor the ability to oversee both shifts, to teach and watch over them as they progressed onto the next level within the company, thus advancing them in their career.

How it was set up prior to my change was basically an industry standard, where there was one day supervisor and one helper on days and one night supervisor and one helper on nights. The day shift worked 6:00 a.m. to 6:00 p.m., and then the night shift worked 6:00 p.m. to 6:00 a.m. The crews usually arrived a little realy for their shift so they can get about a fifteen-minute window on each side to teach the cross shift everything they need to know about what they did for the last 12 hours, what to watch out for, and what they needed to have done. Once a guy reaches the position of a night supervisor, really they need to be self taught to make the next jump, which is really a make or break situation.

My plan made it so one night supervisor and one helper were on one twelve-hour shift, with another night supervisor and helper on the other twelve-hour shift. The shifts would be from 12:00 a.m. to 12:00 p.m., and 12:00 p.m. to 12:00 a.m., but I would leave the day supervisor's schedule the same. he would have to drive himself out to the location alone, as his schedule was from 6:00 a.m. to 6:00 p.m. This was to his benefit, because he could now have the support of the night supervisor to help him ensure the job went smoothly while being able to provide support and training for six hours to each crew. He would also be able to stay longer if things weren't going right, or show up earlier if he wanted to double-check that things were safe for his guys. I also made it so he could leave a little early if things were going smoothly. He could manage his schedule in a way that was more efficient while ensuring the job was on track. If he wanted to spend more time with either crew and provide more training, he could. This gave him the chance to make great improvements and really take ownership of the job.

Really, it ended up being a promotion for not only the little guys but for everyone in the company to have a little more freedom to do the job as they felt fit. When you work with professionals, you need to trust your guys to do what they are good at. So many people don't have enough trust in their employees, and when that happens, things come apart at the seams. That phone call was the eye-opener that I needed to evolve and grow with everyone who was working with me.

Another huge perk was that the day supervisor's truck was also left untouched by new workers/green hands, because we all know new guys typically don't have respect for other people's property and need to be taught. A lot of the times newer workers they don't realize how hard someone has to work to be in a position where they can buy a $70,000 truck, and they don't want it ruined by some kid who decided not to wash the grease off his hands prior to jumping in. In our company/industry, it solved so many problems with this change. Once this change was made, things seemed to run more smoothly as more knowledge was being shared and more training was happening. If the new guys had any questions, they would ask their direct supervisor (night guy) who, for the most part, should be able to answer their questions. But if they were not able to answer them, they could ask the day supervisor during the six-hour shift overlap, thus giving the entire crew the opportunity to learn and advance their career, because everyone had access to the most experienced person on their crew. My guys became the best in the business, and to this day I still believe that!

The night guys were able to spend six hours with the day supervisor to also improve their career skills, which is where we saw the biggest change, and there were no oil spills or injuries reported during that time. This move also made our company the best in the surrounding area, and all it took to make it happen was some intuitive thinking.

It would cost the oil company a little more for a third truck and extra man, but that was a small price to pay to help ensure no recordable injuries or spills occurred. I presented this idea to the oil companies and explained the benefits they would see from it, including that it would cut costs in other areas, like when they needed parts picked up or things delivered, thus cutting the cost of the hot shots to their location.

I remember how it took a lot of juggling to get it all put in place, because this shift had to happen while people were still working, but at midnight on our project launch day, we were ready to make the change! I sat by my phone, ready to field any confusion or issues that may come up during this massive corporate organizational switcho- ver. And you know what? I didn't even receive one call or even a text. It all went like clockwork, and all it took was a lot of thought with proper and exact execution.

Kids, when problems come up, don't look at what's right in front of you. Look at everything, including what could be missing from the big picture.

At this time, there was a marked increase in team collaboration, causing everyone's work ethic and quality of work to improve dra- matically! An oil company even presented me with an innovative thinking and zero incidents award, a trophy to put on my desk that I proudly displayed. Its too bad that when I was let go for having cancer the corporate office felt it best for them to keep it in head office as their accomplishment and not mine, which I guess was OK, but all ll I have to show for it now is a story I can put in this book.

If I'd never gotten that call from my employee, or if I'd decided not to answer it or hang up on him, things would have turned out completely different. He opened my eyes to a growing problem we were facing and got everyone else promoted who deserved a promotion. This really is a true example of the squeaky wheel getting the grease.

Kids, don't be scared to let people know what your true intentions are. Most people are thoughtful and will try to go out of their way to help you. But if you don't show them your determination or express any interest to the ones who can, then no one will ever know to help you. Just like when they had that helicopter job. If I'd spoken up and said I was interested, or that I was the best man for the job, things may have been totally different. You could have had a dad who was a helicopter pilot. But because I was too scared to speak up and say what I felt I deserved, that opportunity slipped by.

I also need to acknowledge my boss around this idea I wanted to try. Without his faith in me and him giving me space to try something I believed in, this would have never happened. Mr. Red, I really am grateful for the trust you had in me.

CHAPTER 26

In The Blink Of An Eye

During the time of my management career, I had more biopsies taken from my tongue. It hurt so much to get a chunk taken out of my already infected/lacerated tongue. You know the pain you get when the dentist drills into a tooth nerve? Think of that on the side of your tongue keeping you in a constant state of pain. You know how much it hurts when you bite into your tongue by accident and it hurts so much you literally stop what ever your doing because of the pain, well think of that pain and have it never go away, that's what I was dealing with. The kind of pain that can bring even the burliest of men to his knees. We had a doctor look at the results in Vancouver and he said it was the stage before cancer (dysplasia) and it wasn't anything serious. Months later, it started to open up even more. It resembled a sideways vagina living on the side of my tongue. If it wasnt a happy vagina that day, it would get angry at me and almost shut me down completely with a pulsating pain throughout my entire body. And every time I ate or drank anything, if any of the fluids or food particles breeched the outside perimeter, it would go into DEFCON 1 mode. It was like there were alarms going off in my body that I never knew I had, and the pain was literally unbearable to the point where I couldn't think of anything else but the pain.

That went on for a bit until I saw a doctor in Edmonton named Dr. Kelsey, and he was a delightful little man. He ordered his tests and, from what I could tell, was not too concerned with what he found. He told me that it was cancer and that he would do a difficult operation, but then he promised me that without a doubt the cancer would be gone. It was funny, because I remember thinking, *You're a doctor—are you allowed to say that you promise you will get all the cancer?* I didn't think that was allowed, because things can change or get misdiagnosed and might not turn out as planned.

For me, finding out I had cancer was like finding out your car needs a major overhaul or expensive repairs. (Now, please note that this is only how *I* felt at the time and place, and it in no way speaks for the experience of anyone else suffering from this horrible disease.) When I was told I had cancer, I was thinking, *Of course it's the worst possible outcome.* Then immediately after that I wondered, *How long will I be off work?* For me, work was the most important thing in my life. I'd like to say it was my wife and kids, but that wasn't how I prioritized things.

In my mind, money gets you what you want, like an education, experiences, and a life you truly want. If you want to try skydiving, you need money. If you want to send your kids to private school, you need money. If you want to eat your next meal, you need money. If you want to own a boat and create priceless memories for the family, you need money. Sorry, babe, I'm not giving up on the buying-a-boat idea!

I worked all the time and even harder when I was at home on days off. I needed to ensure my family was financially secure and that they could have the freedom to do whatever they wanted (minus me, if I was away at the time, which was basically all the time), and I wanted to make sure they had everything they could ever want or need—financially speaking, of course.

Before the cancer and after, while I still had a job, I worked my ass off to own property like my dad did, by this point I had three houses—two in Red Deer and one in Sylvan Lake. Also, I purchased a half acre of land in Anglemont, BC, where we were able to take vacations with our massive camper that we pulled behind my new Dodge Ram 3500 dually truck. We also owned a van for my wife to transport the kids, and a kick-ass sports car that I believe I mention later in the book, which was a gleaming silver 2000 Pontiac Trans Am in mint condition!

So the news of the cancer came along and I was thinking, *How this will affect my career?* The first person I told beside my immediate family members was Mr. Red, who assured me that if I couldn't continue to do my job as a manager, they would find another position where I could continue employment, and he would ensure I was always employed. Telling my boss was a humbling experience, but it was when I told others that I saw more distant family and friends starting to pull away. Sadly, after all my surgeries, my new financial burden overcame us, and we had to sell off everything.

At that time I was extremely depressed, to say the least. The reality of my situation was setting in, and I was losing so much in my life— I lost the way I looked, sounded and acted, I even lost the way I walked. Everything was changing, and it was like the world was rapidly forgetting about us and leaving me and my family behind to waste away. I wish I had better words to explain the loneliness I felt in this situation, and the words that really explained the impact this all had on my wife and kids. I pray that no one ever has to feel like that, as it's the worst feeling anyone can have. The expression of helplessness, abandonment and loneliness doesn't even come close to how we all actually felt.

If this has ever happened to you, then you know. But if it hasn't, the best way I can explain it is like this:

It's like when you were a young kid on a packed bus with your daycare group. The bus makes its normal stop, and everyone in the group gets off, though you don't notice, and the bus continues on its route. The bus has gone a few more stops before you realize you are all alone, and you are way too far away to be able to go back on your own. You are lost and confused and scared and just devastated that this has happened to you. You are completely alone , scared, and for the first time in your life you are actually lost. You must make a choice here, but every choice has outcomes that will make things even harder. Regardless of what choice you make, you will have a difficult road ahead. That's the feeling right here. It is devastating and soul-crushing.

Instantly, you are on that bus by yourself, so you can be sad and cry to yourself or be mad—for me, there were no ifs, ands, or buts about it—I was fucking mad.

First option: You hit the stop bell now and walk back to your people. That's a hell of a trek on your own, but it's doable. You just need to be committed to the uphill battle. Do I figure this all out on my own and act like nothing happened, hide my fears, and walk on my own, while everyone else just goes on with their lives and never even looks back at me?

Second option: Be embarrassed and tell the bus driver you missed your stop. The people on the bus will be mad that the bus has to turn around. They just want life to continue, regardless of whether you're at the right stop. Some people on the bus might be happy you're going back to where you are safe, but you're putting all your trust in a total stranger and hoping he is good enough to know exactly where your stop should be. All my trust was in the surgeon/bus driver to get me back to where I should be.

Third option: Ride the bus to the end and hope for the best. There, people wouldn't even know you were there. Some would approach you to see if you were OK because you were obviously alone. (This signifies the people that can see I am in need but am too proud to ask for help. They do what they can to help.)

Well, I got to try all three options. First, I tried option three, where I just wanted to ride the bus and didn't care that I had cancer. I just wanted to continue with life and hope to God that my problem got magically solved. Well, that didn't happen, so I felt confused, frustrated, and of course still angry at myself. Some people showed some concern for me here, but most didn't.

Then I chose option two, where I pissed off a lot of people, but when we got to the stop that the bus driver felt was mine, some people felt I was wasting time in their more-than-important lives, some were happy I made it to my stop, and some got off the bus with me to ensure that it was my stop. But most didn't. Kind of like how my doctor finished up the surgery and said, "That's it; it's all done and over with, and I can't do anything more for you. You are on your own."

Then, because it was not my actual stop, I had only one option left. So I picked option one, but with a twist. Those few people that got off the bus with me who really cared about me and my family started that long walk back with me to the right stop, where my group had gotten off the bus. Here was where, for the first time, I did not feel anger. I was grateful to know who my real family (only half of whom are blood related) were. It's all those who ensured I not only got off at the bus stop but walked with me on that huge journey that I seemed to pass right by.

CHAPTER 27

Red Lobster

Basically, as soon as it was determined that I had cancer and they were going to operate, we scheduled a surgery to remove half my tongue. I really didn't know what to expect, but I was ready for anything. Honestly, to me, it was like I was going to go on a business trip and didn't know when I was going to come back. People made such a big deal about it, and I didn't really understand why. I was just having a surgery. Surgeries happen every day to all kinds of people, so what was the big fucking deal?? But to play along, I decided that my wife and I would go for my last *real* meal before the day of surgery.

Where would you go? We went to Red Lobster in Edmonton! (mmmmmm) My last meal was lobster bisque. Now, really think of that: if you were to only have one meal left in your life that you could taste, where would you go?

To you guys at Red Lobster, this is a huge compliment, because that was my last real meal in life, and I wanted to eat there. Maybe I could do a commercial for Red Lobster one day stating that the food is so good it's to die for. (Would that be too cheesy?) I have many ideas about how we could do these commercials. I could dress up like a lobster, looking all shriveled and sickly, and we could have a healthy one played by someone like the Rock, looking all healthy and strong. Then we both pretend to be caught in a lobster trap, and I turn to the Rock, who is of course dressed as a rock lobster (Get it? *Rock* lobster? Lol) and say, "Well, at least we will die making someone happy," and he could say, "No, not you, my friend. You will not make it through tonight's lobster selection." Then one of the fishermen throws me back. Then you see the Rock getting lowered into a pot of boiling water as he says, "Can you smell what the Rock is cooking?"

OK, maybe not. Maybe that's kind of stupid ... or is it??? Guess we will find out if Red Lobster contacts me to do a commercial.

But in all seriousness, because we didn't have Red Lobster in our city, it was a really special thing when we decided to go there. It basically was a full day planned around eating at their restaurant because of the travel time it took to get there.

But the funny thing about my last meal, the lobster bisque, was that it is probably the thing I like least on their menu. I have always found that lobster bisque tastes like ground-up lobster shell and ocean floor mixed together—but that's just my opinion. I would have preferred to eat their actual lobster and steak or crab, which is why I picked the place. I like the idea of being presented with such amazing seafood that smells so good. And my wife also loves it there! Personally, I think crab gets overlooked a lot and that it outweighs the lobster when it comes to flavor. Everyone always makes big stink when it comes to lobster—and rightfully so, as lobster is an amazing food. I mean, hell, it's a food that when you are on a date and she orders it, it makes you think: *Holy shit, she ordered the lobster! I'm getting laid!* Now if that doesn't say it's one amazing food, I don't know what does. I believe lobster is a super food, but if you were to truly have a taste test and put lobster against crab, I'm sure the crab would win, hands down every time!

Sorry, I got sidetracked. But the reason I had the bisque was because I couldn't eat anything solid. The pain solid food would inflict on me was so terrible and unbearable. If I ate anything more solid, it would rub inside the sideways, vagina-shaped, cottage-cheese-filled infection that was taking over my tongue. Oh, and the pain. It was un-fucking bearable, total unimaginable pain, even when eating the soup. This is also why I was losing weight so drastically. I was 177 pounds before the cancer and 101 pounds at my lowest point. Prior to this and for the pain, I was prescribed Oxycodone while waiting for surgery, and I was popping those like candy. I kept increasing my dosages because my body kept developing an immunity to it, so obviously I was addicted to this drug and would have insane with drawls in forms of very nasty temper tantrums if I didn't have the pills on a a very regular basis. I was quite literally angry all the time, even during the times I didn't appear to be. I was one very pissed-off cancer victim! I was mad at everyone and took it out on most of the people I knew and loved. This is also probably why I lost most of my friends and family. I used to think it was because they didn't want to be around a sick person, but I probably drove them all away with how angry I was. My advice to you is that if you are caring for someone you love and have to face their anger and frustration directly, know this: people will often take it out on their loved ones the most. They know that they don't have to worry as much about how they are perceived and can be themselves, and if being angry is how they cope with it, then you need to try your best to work your way through it with them. I took it out on my loved ones because I felt they needed to share my pain.

OK, back to the restaurant. Here I was sitting at the table with Bambi awaiting my bisque. To me, it was the perfect last meal, because lobster is a good choice as a last meal—well, at least according to movies for guys on death row. and for me, my last meal was some kind of liquified food that would be somewhat easier to rinse out of the cottage-cheese-filled vagina growing inside my mouth.

After our supper, we headed to the hotel to sleep, as surgery was happening the very next morning.

CHAPTER 28

Pain And Suffering

We arrived at the hospital, and I was told that I was going to be put under anaesthetic for eighteen hours. But I wasn't worried at all. I was never scared about the surgery—in fact, it was the opposite. I had only ever been under a general anaesthetic once before, and what I remember about waking up was a feeling of amazingness. It was probably the drugs, but I still remember never feeling more hydrated, refreshed, and well rested in my life. So I was looking forward to that feeling again. It was like a messenger came down from the sky and offered me a small piece of heaven as I woke up, like a heavenly messenger! Funny, I don't remember if I really cared so much about removing the cancer, but I recall that I was craving the opportunity to have an amazing wake-up experience! So I was actually kind of excited to get to the surgery so I could feel that again. Please remember I had lived with that terrible pain for a few years by this point and waking up not in pain was something I had been craving for such a long time.

The eighteen hours came and went, and I was starting to open my eyes, ready for this amazing feeling of tranquility. But, HELL NO! It was complete and utter fucking pain. Nothing like the pain I had before. It penetrated through both flesh and bone. Hell, I could even feel it through my eyes! I woke up with every pain receptacle in my body raging, as if I was awake while my body was going through a meat grinder. It was the worst fucking pain I ever experienced in my entire life—in fact, in both yours and my life combined. It was literally like I was fully awake during the middle of my surgery.

All I could think was, *Kill me, kill me now, holy fucking fuck, PLEASE KILL ME NOW! I need something to end this pain, be it more drugs or a bullet, I don't care.* I remember thinking, *Please, Lord, I beg of you, please call on the power of lightning and have it strike straight through my soul and explode my body into a billion pieces of nothingness. I was like nothing I had ever felt or even imagined that I would feel, like the pain of someone that got wounded in a fierce battle or mauled by a lion*

GUESS WHAT WE FOUND OUT THAT DAY. We found out that a small percentage of people do not feel the effects of morphine. And guess who is one of those people? ARE YOU FUCKING KIDDING ME? For fuck's sake, I felt the excruciating pain of having half my tongue removed, the five-by-four-inch chunk of flesh and muscle they took from my left arm to replace the half of my tongue they took from my face, and the massive skin graft they removed from my left leg to cover and stitch into my left arm to cover the gaping chunk they removed. Let alone the new feeling of the trachea they installed into my throat, as well as the incision they needed to make from ear lobe to ear lobe across my entire throat to get access to the far back of my tongue to do the incisions. They also removed all my thyroid glands in the process.

Here is a small tip if you are going in for a major surgery and they plan on putting you on the morphine drip: maybe see if they can find out *prior* to the surgery if it will work for you. I don't know if they can test for that, but it sure wouldn't hurt to ask. I know I wish I did.

But once we solved that, by almost doubling the oxy dosage I was taking prior to this, the pain was a lot more bearable, and it was smooth sailing for what could be expected. To be honest, even to this day I am disappointed that I didn't get my heavenly wake-up.

But all in all, the surgery was successful and, to be honest, it was the best I could hope for, so I thought.

So there I was in STAGE 2, recovering from surgery.

CHAPTER 29

I'm Only A File Number

As I write this part, I feel a sense of sadness and here's why. During this time, I had many follow up appointments with rehab, speech pathologists, reconstructive surgeons, nurses, and doctors. There were people coming and going to my hospital room at all hours of the day and night. There were nurses who were so mean and nurses who made the sun shine so brightly in your window-less room that you had to put sunglasses on. The process of healing was long and challenging. What the doctor was able to do during this surgery was pretty remarkable when you think about it. They removed literally half my tongue and cut what I can only describe as what looked like a shark bite from my forearm. I have an oval-shaped scar on my left forearm now where they removed about a five-inch-long section. They then folded that in half and sewed it onto the living/good side of my tongue, which I could only imagine was a bloody mess in my mouth. Then they took a skin graft from my left leg and covered the shark bite on my arm and sewed it all up. When I woke up, there were hoses and tubes sticking out of me and pumps and beeping things all over. I ended up getting a massive bedsore just above my ass. My body was covered in well over 100 staples, lots and lots of stitches, new holes, and tons of scabs.

But the good news was that my tongue did not hurt at all. I mean, it hurt, but not in the same way as it did before the surgery. And during this journey, I was to meet two amazing people who would turn into long-term friends.

In my hospital room I had more than one roommate during my stay, which was actually lucky. The room mates drastically helped with sanity and human connection, because every doctor nurse and staff member treated you as just a file number. But out of all the roommates I had over the months of recovery, there was one guy Mike, who was probably the most amazing man I will ever meet. Mike had a different kind of cancer—I believe it was in this throat and voice box. We never really discussed his cancer or mine, probably for two reasons. One was that we both came from the same upbringing, where you don't really express your feelings or problems. The other and probably more realistic reason was neither of us could talk. I had half a tongue and he had no voice box. But make no mistake: Mike didn't ever skip a beat. In fact, he was usually the one to cause the beat! A good-looking nurse would walk in, he would grab her by the hand, and next thing you knew, a disco fever dance party broke out right in front of me. This man was larger than life! He and I would communicate with facial expressions and hand gestures. When my trachea was removed (for the first time) and I was able to make noises again, I was able to talk to him in my slurred speech. Between his and my stubbornness, we were able to make the best of the situation we were in. Unfortunately, he died from his cancer, as so many do from this horrible disease, but I am so proud I had the privilege to meet him and become friends with him and his amazing wife, Amy.

Amy lost her husband to cancer, but he fought a great battle. To me, Mike was a guy who knew how he wanted to live, and he is a hero in my eyes. While we were in the hospital, I made a promise to Mike that one day we would sit down and have our first beer together and look back at this shit and laugh. We did have some good laughs together, but sadly, not the beer. But as a man of my word, when I recovered enough, my family and I had the chance to visit his farm, where we all sat together with his urn in the middle of the table. And with both our families present, we all enjoyed a beer together, as promised. His grandkids and my kids joined us with a root beer.

I toasted him by saying "Hey, Mike, I didn't think you would literally be on the table when we drank, but I am glad we finally did get that drink together. And I promise that I will use the rest of my life to make an impact in peoples lives in any way I can "

To get released from the hospitals grasp, I had to endure thirty-three rounds of radiation, three rounds of intense chemo and every test you could possibly imagine . The worst decision I made during all of this was that after many, many months of using oxy as a pain-killer, I decided that the first day of chemo was a great time to stop it using it altogether. YEAH, THAT WAS STUPID. I didn't have any pain in my tongue now, so I didn't think I would need it anymore. I don't recall anyone advising me that I needed to ween myself off it, so the day I was to have my first round of chemo, I stopped cold-ass turkey and almost killed myself and put my stupid ass back in the hospitals intensive care unit! Not only was my body receiving this foreign drug forced into its system, but I made the decision to take the one thing away that it craved, and thought it relied on. Those were the roughest couple of days I ever had to overcome in my life! I didn't clue in to why my body was shutting down and just assumed it was the chemo.

Only now do I understand when people say that it's an extremely hard addiction to break. Too bad I wasn't informed enough to put that together—way to go, you dumb shit. But that was no one's fault but my own, Sorry, Mom and Bambi, for scaring you two like that, but thank you so much for staying at my side the whole time I was going through it!

There is more to the story on why I chose to quit that day, not only did I know the tongue pain was gone, there was an incident that happened the night before what made me decide it was totally necessary. At the time I don't even recall this happening but I was told this that morning and there was proof that this terrifying experience did actually happen.

That morning I woke up like every morning where my body was cold and sweaty craving my drug, but this particular morning I also woke up to my wife very upset with me, so much that she demanded an apology for my actions that night. Not recalling anything out of the ordinary I was very quick to tell her I have nothing to apologize for. She then went on to tell me that not only was I yelling at my kids for not eating supper fast enough and not thanking me for making supper (which she assures me they did), she tells me that I had a complete melt down over this and smashed their plates on the dinner table and threw a fork at her in my moment of rage. Knowing I would never do this , let lone would not remember something like this from the night before I told her "You're fucked" and scrambled down to the kitchen to get my pills. When I got to the kitchen I couldn't believe my eyes, there were broken plates and food that had no place being where it was. She clearly was not telling a lie, and I was completely caught off guard that this actually happened and I had no fucking recollection or it at all.

So nedless to say, I decided to quit cold turkey immediately as I never wanted my family to not feel safe especially when they are at home.

But regardless of the crappy decision on timing I did make it through and I did get through the chemo and radiation, which I have to say was the absolute worst thing my body ever went through. This is just how radiation affected me, but from my experience, I would recommend not getting the radiation if you don't have to. Radiation is like a cancer all its own, one that will slowly keep on fucking you up even long after you are actually considered healthy. It feels like your body is literally drying up and taking every bit of energy you have. The feeling lasts between treatments and doesn't go away; it's the gift that keeps on giving.

A few months went by and we all thought this was the last of the cancer! By this point, I still didn't truly feel like I was ever dying of cancer, more a feeling like I was sick with a cold that put me out of commission for a long time, I thought it was something that will pass over time. By this point, I always knew I was "easily" going to get through this; it was all just a matter of time, more of a waiting game, but I knew I was going to get through it in the end. Don't get me wrong, I did have many moments of weakness where my head would go into a freak out what if game, (kind of like you do when you dream of winning the lottery, where your brain sets you off to some imaginary dream land where you won billions. Those times were just like that , but way way more morbid. Those were always scary but I would come back to the real world and know that was never going to happen to me, I will not die from this. The statistics are in my favour as we caught in time, as I was assured by our doctors. My only real fear that I knew I would have to actually face were mostly fears based around how I was going to talk with half a tongue and get through life sounding disabled person. That was my biggest fear back then.

During this time of recovery and being basically bedridden, you realize that your life has come to an abrupt halt, and you realize that everyone's life around you keeps on going and moving forward! You watch people come to work, and punch out then to act like another person. You realize that you become someone's job, and they see many people just like you where they say the same things to each of us , like a story about their drive to work. They may tell it 20 times that day just to make small talk. You have no friends there or people you can really rely on to understand what you are going through. They didn't care what would happen to me , they just needed me well enough to free up the bed to bring on the next job to get completed. Like a back up in the logging yard, get it in and processed and get it the fuck out of here. You lay there and watch your loved ones' eyes blacken as they watch you almost lifeless. So that was the time I had to grasp on to anything that was positive to inspire me try to keep going. I had to do whatever I could to have just one more day with my family and to beat this thing. The one thing that gave me some hope was that I was still employed, so when I was feeling up to it, I devoted all my time to working as much as I possibly could. I would do anything and everything in my power to build a future for my wife and kids, so my goal was to prove to the president of the company that, despite the shit I was going through, I could continue to do an exceptional job for them. I knew I would live through this, but I had to make sure I had a job when I did, so like a good man would I worked my ass off to make sure I still was the bread maker for my family's financial stability. I was hell bent on showing them that I was a key part of this company.

So I focused all my energy on keeping files organized and up to date, filling in spreadsheets, and collecting stats. I made sure that I rested when I needed to and watched movies when my mind needed a break, but mainly my focus was on that laptop, doing everything I could to ensure everything within my department ran smoothly, which I am proud to say worked out just fine. After I was mostly recovered from that harsh surgery, I was able to go on a work trip to Florida to gather information on some of the newest technologies that were being presented at an oil and gas conference. I was kicking ass and taking names and didn't want to fall behind on anything.

After about three months had passed since my surgery, and my routine CT scan showed us all the cancer was non existent, and we all knew the worst had past and it was basically over with. But not even two weeks after that scan was completed. I started developing an open sore on the inside and outside of both my cheeks—I had it checked out, and the doctor said that it was decaying tissue about the size of an American quarter forming on both sides my face. So they took a biopsy and, sure as shit, it was cancer.

They scheduled me in right away for a CT scan, and it felt as though everything happened too quickly. The next thing I knew, we were discussing how the doctors would have to cut out more of my tongue and would have to remove more chunks out of various areas of my body to fill that gap in my mouth. And how in the next couple of days, I would be feeding myself through a tube that went up my nose and down directly into my stomach, instead of eating like a baby bird that tilts its head back and waits for the food to slide down its throat, which is what I had been doing. Not to mention that I would probably not be able to talk to my kids ever again. Literally that morning I had been talking about getting back to work on my regular twenty-and-ten rotation, and here I was a few hours later, being told that I would now never be able to talk again. This is not how I envisioned that day would go when I woke up that morning. The doctor then proceeded to tell me that we would be heading in for surgery within the next few days, and to be prepared to be stuck in the hospital for many many months during recovery.

So after having received two completely good test results stating that the cancer was for sure gone, I was heading back in for surgery because the cancer had exploded and was all over my body, including the base of my skull and into my lungs. Basically, I was littered with it. Without any indication or warning signs, the cancer had decided to get fully aggressive and spread all over. We were later told that the surgeon Made an error the first time and because he didn't get the right margins, it agitated it and spread like wild fire. This after I was told it was totally gone and not to worry. That was the hardest roller-coaster of emotions that we all had to over come, and overcome very quickly. Because we only had days to prepare for me to be away from home for up to 6 months and get everything re-planned out where my support system is there for me again. It fucked up a lot of my friends and families lives up. They had that task to come visit me on a weekly basis or bi weekly bases depending how far away they lived.

CHAPTER 30

Third and Fourth-String Surgeons

A couple of days went by after receiving the new diagnosis, and I arrived at the hospital to undergo surgery #2. This time it was expected to take about twenty-two to twenty- four hours, which to me seemed to be about the norm by this point.

In I went for even more removal of my 1/2 tongue, which also included the total removal of the new ½ piece they'd already added from my arm. They were planning on taking another quarter of my tongue. There was a slight hope I would still be able to talk, but I figured there was probably no more talking for this cowboy. Still, I never did feel sad for myself. I just thought, *Well, this will be different.*

Like after the first surgery, I assumed I would wake up with large bedsores on my legs and around my tail bone. But I hoped after this one knowing what we know about Morphine, I would wake up in that state of feeling great. I don't know what the hell happened, but I awoke from the second surgery with tubes, monitors, wires, and rubber things sticking out all over me. I was mortified at what I was looking at. I was looking at my newly stitched-up body parts, which were covered by blood-soaked bandages, I knew something hadn't gone as planned. The skills and workmanship of the surgeons were less than sub-par this time. I don't know who was working onme , but it was like that tattoo artist that didn't know how to draw. All I could think was it had to be a situation where its like having a football team losing so badly you decide to send in the third-string just so they could say they got to play in a game. That's exactly what happened. I remembered thinking I looked like I was in a bad motorcycle accident, traveling at a high speed and wearing nothing but shorts and a T-shirt. I looked like a third grader's model clay project of their interpretation of abstract art. I didn't expect to wake up with a face so distorted, and a body to match.

The surgery did not go as planned, as the doctors made an executive decision and removed the entire tongue, not just three-quarters of it like they had planned. They also discovered cancer in my jawbone, so they had to remove three quarters of my lower jaw. They literally removed the lower part of my face. They couldn't leave me without a lower jaw, so they cut into my left leg and removed my fibula, which they somehow broke apart and turned into what is now my lower jawbone. For those of you who are like me and had no idea what bone that is, it's the bone parallel to your shinbone. Apparently, there are two bones in the lower half of your leg—I didn't know that. So I didn't lose a bone but that I had a backup jaw that I never knew I had right here, tucked away in my left leg. I even have a spare in my right leg now, just in case I ever need it!

So my new reality was that I had to learn how to walk again, talk again or find some way of easy communication opposed to always having to text, eat again through my new stomach tube that hangs out over two feet long, and breathe again, because of course I had a new trachea installed. It was like starting from scratch all over, but this time remembering every heart-ache along the way un-like how a baby forgets This was going to be my hardest struggle in my life and I knew it wasn't going to be fun . I also had to learn to communicate with my kids, who couldn't read as of yet. I imagine waking up in total shock and realizing that you have no way to communicate with your kids.

I also had to learn how to sleep. (It wasn't even something that I thought I had to consider, but when you have tubes and hoses and things all attached to you, it's not like sleeping is easy when you can't lay in certain positions you're used to). I had to re-learn how to use the washroom. When I was in the hospital, I literally had to shit in a plastic pan in my bed. Believe it or not, through all that, I was still able to work and do my job the same as I had before the surgeries. My work was strictly computer based, so I was able to do it all from a hospital bed.

I remember one specific terrible moment during my recovery stage. I was going for a walk and was walking very slowly. I was still very weak, as I still had many more months of recovery ahead of me, and Bambi was walking about in front of me when all of a sudden I just broke down in tears. It ripped my heart to shreds, and I felt like a complete failure because she was walking faster, and even with all the strength I had, I couldn't keep up to her. I felt like she had to be so disappointed in me, and I was trying so hard to walk beside my wife, but she was just about three feet in front of me. But I couldn't do it. Even to this day when I think about this it brings tears to my eyes, and I have to admit it hurts my heart so much to even think about it. I just want to curl up and cry again.

That was the worst feeling ever, to feel like I was letting down the only person I wanted so desperately to make proud. Bambi was the only one I could count on to be there for me every day and to push me to work harder and never give up, but she would also always catch me when I fell. Letting her down felt worse than lying in a bed dying, feeling utterly and completely hopeless to the world. This moment in my life impacted me more than any other time during this journey, when I knew I had to push myself, regardless of everything, as I didn't ever want my wife to have to see me let her down again.

Through Her Eyes (Bambi's notes, unedited)

Has small resin on tongue when I was in dental assisting school. Went to mall ads to have teeth checked before I went into school in 2005.

Did school.
Found out that if things didn't heal in 14 days then this was no usual.

Started work in 2007 at mall dental office.
Did check-up on Jason around when Zack was born, 2009 b/c lesion on tongue was not healing or was back.

Went to Dr. N in Red Deer and had a biopsy taken. Results came back negative.

Things healed for the most part. Jason went back to work in US.

The year 2011 bought Jason a car for five-year anniversary present. In 2011 in Vancouver, tongue was still hurting, has another biopsy done in Vancouver
Results not given but found out later that the result were precancerous.

In 2012, went back to Dr. H in Red Deer for another biopsy as was referred by Dr. Z in the mall because lesion was starting to cause pain and was not healing.

Results came back nothing there.
End of 2012 went back again and demanded another biopsy b/c it was very painful, and Bambi could not deal with how grouchy Jason had

become, and so she demanded that another biopsy be taken. Another biopsy was taken at Dr. H's office. Stage 4 cancer result was given.

Went to Edmonton and had first surgery
November 5, 2013.

In Edmonton have second surgery July 9, 2014

July 9, 2 a.m.
Well, Jason's out. He's very much awake compared to last time. He's coherent enough to ask me not to leave him and write I love you on my hand. He also gave me the Kom-Tong stare. He's not in any pain. They did remove his entire jaw bone. And all of his tongue. He does not know about his tongue yet and he will be upset. But Dr. S thought it was best just to take it all out. They used his fibula for his new jaw bone and muscle and skin from that area and his upper thigh for replacing his skin under his mouth. I have asked that they put him in his side so that he won't get a bed sore this time. It's very hard seeing him like this but thankfully I did not cry in front of him. Like I said, he is very aware of where he is and who he is and what he had done. They won't let me back in the unit tonight. They said he's been awake since 1:10 am when they moved him to the burn unit. So they have him done Dilotted to help him sleep. I am able to go back in the morning, so I will update you guys then.
July 9, 10:30
Dad and I came to the hospital in unit 3c2 to see you u. this is the burn unit. You told me to extend my hotel for 10 days. You also wrote for me and dad to talk because you liked listening. Our nurses name is "glide the letter." He is very nice. He was a little chatterbox this morning and asked lots of questions and laughed and joked around. Very nice guy.

So today is a little worse for Jason. He's in a bit of pain. He says mostly in his leg. They tried to switch him over to cold air breathing in his own. He was not having it. I don't know if you remember, but last time he had a collapsed lung. With fluid in it. He had to have a few x rays. I really hope that him not switching over to the cold air doesn't make it worse in the long run. I asked the respiratory nurse. But she said it should be ok for now. She will try again later.

11:05 a.m.
The unit head nurse just came in. She is worried that Jason didn't switch over to the cold air flow. She wants to get an X-ray of his lungs. The longer he is on the warm air flow the more likely he will develop pneumonia. He says his pain level is a 7 or 8. She says with his history of cancer he is at a higher percentage to develop blood clots and get clots in his lungs if he doesn't switch over or sit up soon. She is getting an X-ray in half an hour and she said she is going to be very firm and if the x ray looks good she will force him onto the cold air breathing machine. She also wants him to sit up and move around a bit more. We will see what the next hour brings.

12 p.m.
Sat up to take -Xray. X-ray looks good. No fluid. Kept Jason sitting up for a bit. Dad and I were in the room when all of a sudden, your eyes went big. And you sat further up and leaned a bit forward. Then you vomited. Everywhere. Dad was really scared but just kept saying to himself keep calm. Ran outside to grab nurse. He cleaned you up. Said "We'll that woke him up, didn't it?" About twenty minutes later you vomited again.

3 p.m.
Sat on the bed for about half an hour, 2:30-3. Wobbled onto chair beside the bed. Foot hurts. Has to have it elevated. Almost ended up

moved to chair by himself. G just was there for balance. He didn't like to be moved. Slammed his fist onto chair arm. Settled watching the Netherlands and Argentina play soccer.

4pm.
Jason's ICU roommate gets moved. Maria. She is missing both her legs. From the knees down. Seemed like a nice lady.

4:15
Dr. S came in to talk about surgery with you. They used all thigh muscles for your new tongue and took out arm part. You just found out he took your whole tongue. You are very worried about talking.

4:30
Got some antibiotics and hep shot. You hate that, but it helps thin the blood clots. Still sitting in chair.

5:15. Moved back to bed. You did it mostly on your own. But when you move you feel sick still. Needed to have bucket. But didn't vomit. Shaking really bad. Freezing cold. You are so tired. You need to rest.

7 p.m.
Shift change. You have a female night nurse. Didn't catch her name. You need to stay in ICU again tonight so they can keep an eye on you. You say you are in a lot of pain still. You are in bed but sitting up watching love it or list it.

7:30
Respiratory nurse came in. Checked vitals and said not to use the suction inside the mouth because of the flaps inside. She asked if I was your mom...... She said sorry. I guess u look young right?! The

night nurse is giving you gravel for your upset tummy. They might try new pain medicine soon.

8:17.

Night nurse doesn't have a name tag. She just told me they forgot to feed you today.

I have two hours of sleep since 4 a.m. I'm not feeling tired yet. I just tossed and turned last night so hopefully I'm tired enough to sleep tonight. Jason is getting drowsy but says I can't leave. Is it done soon? Maybe I can let Jason hear his kids voices! That might be cool. Kids called but you were pretty out of it. Hopefully tomorrow :)

10pm

Night nurse told me that I should get some rest. She promised that she would keep a very close eye on you. She seems honest. She has been coming in every hour. So I went home.

July 10

Day nurse's name is Amanda.

She had already had you sitting up in a chair for an hour and had just moved you back into bed when I came at 10 am. The pain medicine is finally starting to work. You are at a six today. Amanda took out the artery IV. It goes directly into your artery. She needed to put pressure on it for five minutes. When she moved you back into bed you felt nauseous and she gave you something for that. So far today you have not thrown up. Your face looks a little more swollen, but you neck looks less swollen.

11am

You got a new roommate named Sammy. They had to move the bed all around and the nurse Erin pulled your nose tube pretty hard. You didn't like it. Then the other nurse made your bed shorter and it hit your bad leg.

11:10.
You just asked for your phone. One day out of surgery. But I left it at the hotel. You are mad.

12 p.m.
You checked Facebook on my phone. You seemed happier. I talked to Mr. Red and told him you were doing good. Didn't tell him you don't have a tongue. Moving still makes you sick. But you pushed your own button on the bed to sit up.

Tiny steps ~ yet so big.

2:30
You have been sleeping for about an hour and a half. You were dreaming about half an hour ago your eyes were just moving around lol. Watching the food network with you made me very hungry and I told the nurse I was thinking of sneaking out but was afraid you would get mad if I came back and you noticed I was gone. But you were still kind of awake then (1pm) and you shook your head no. You wouldn't be mad. So I went and tried a turkey burger and fries. It was ok. Was back at 1:15. You were sleeping. Nurse added phosphorous. She said your levels were low. The other ladies nurse isn't as nice as ours. She is probably tired. She's kind of snotty when she asks me to move, pluses she keeps pulling on your nose tube and waking you up because she is moving her patient in and out of the chair and she moves your nose feed way out of the way. I hope she's done now. You said your pain is at a five. Yay!!! It's coming down. You for sure do not want to hold my hand or want me to hold your hand. I hope your just sore and not mad at me. It's hard to know because you can't talk yet.

3:30.

You got moved to 3d4. Room 34.

Very upset as this room has no tv. I said I could read to you. You said no. I said I could sing to you. You said no. You wrote for me to get the phone and computer. So that you have something to do. Our new nurses name is Pam. She is in until 11pm. Your pain has gone down to a 5. So that's good. This room is boring.

3:40

Tara and Adrien sent some flowers for you. They are in a boot. Cute!!

4pm

You keep motioning for me to get your phone. I give in. I'll go in rush hour traffic to give in. I'll go in rush hour traffic to get your stupid phone.

And computer.

6:15

We set up computer and watch Talladega nights.

About 7 p.m., three quarters of through the movie you decided you need to poo

Got the Nurse but they don't want you to use toilet do they got a little bedpan thing for you. Boy, is it uncomfortable. Took twenty minutes to get you positioned on there and right near the end Mike knocked on the door. We made him wait. You farted, and I took the bedpan away. They visited for about fifteen minutes or so. Then they left. After they left, you felt very hot. We took the blankets off—that didn't help. So I got the nurse. She was taking forever and suctioned out your tube. Then another forever before she got your gravel. The respiratory nurse came in and you coughed up a huge phlegm blood clot thing.

Mike and Amy, his wife, came to visit. They only stayed ten minutes.

8:45
Kids called. You didn't want to listen to them, so I left the room and chatted with them. Your sister bought Kisenya a new bike and new running shoes, and your mom bought them new back packs and Zack a new pair of swim trunks. No wonder they like going there ;) they are having fun though. They went to the library and went swimming and rode their bones today. Yesterday they went exploring and watered plants and walked the dogs.

10:45
New night nurse.
Jims. He was here before, nice guy. Tattoos on left arm. Did vitals. Gave you shot. You are at a 5 for pain. We decided to watch the last little bit if Talladega nights.

11:15.
You feel hot.
Took all blankets off and readjusted you. You are starting to get a bed sore.

11:30
Still hot. I got the nurse. He gave us done wet clothes to put on you. You said you just want to be normal again. "Just get me normal again."

12:45
I try to sleep, but you feel really sick. You think you are going to vomit. You do. And you say it really burns. I got the inner cannula out and got one of the nurses. She didn't do anything. The respiratory nurse and I try to clean you up. She suctions you. She gets a small blood clot out. You have vomit and a ton of blood coming out of your mouth and nose. It's scary. I try to stay calm. And also, not to vomit. It's hard. I

gag once. Vomit is all in your mouth. I get the green stick things and chlorhexidine to try to freshen your mouth and to get the burning out. The nurse finds you something for nausea. You say you hate this food because it makes you sick. And that it burns in your nose and mouth. Shitty. One step forward. 2 back.

3-4 a.m. you wrote a note saying it still burns. The vomit hurts the back of your throat.
6am. You feel like you have to poop. Nothing again.

6:30
Dr. S, a resident, looks at you. He says everything looks and sounds good. He wants to take the balloon in your throat down. And get you off the press your own button pain medication. I think they will probably put you on oxy.
You tell me you are cold and a little ill. We get you Gravol.

7:20
Day nurse comes on. Takes vitals.
So many nurses coming and going.
Jason had a rough night. His days and nights are mixed up so he was up most of the night. Plus the food they are giving him makes him nauseous and he threw up. Then for five-and-a-half hours he kept telling me and the nurses how much it burned. Unfortunately, there is absolutely nothing they can do. I washed his mouth put and his face all up. The nurse last night was useless. Of course, when he vomits it scares him and makes him feel like he can't breathe. I took the trachea out so he could catch his breath.

This morning the dr came In and said he wants to take Jason off the pain button and deflate the balloon in his trachea. A bit scary cause if he throws up again it can get into his lungs now. But good because it's one step closer to getting the trachea out. We turned the food off until the dietician comes in. He hated this food, and last time they switched Him to something different.

Positive step this morning is that he went all the way around the ward with the help of the girl physiotherapists, and they let him go at his own pace. I reminded him to take his time and he did. He took too breaks and did fine. He feels a bit nauseated from getting up and moving but he did amazing. I am so so proud of him. Now he's getting a sponge bath. He has to sit up in the chair for an hour or more today before he can go back into his bed. The physiotherapists will be back again this afternoon to take him around again. It's a bit harder this time because they want him up and moving around, but they don't want him to put weight on his one leg. That means that him and I can't go for a walk like we had initially planned. Most of the nurses and secrets and residents remember him from last time, and it's nice to see a few friendly faces. I feel bad because the nurse knows my name, but I have no clue what hers is.

Her name is Kane. She has a fourteen-year-old daughter. And our nurse who cleans the beds and sponges Jason is Carmen.

1:10
Got cleaned up. Got Oxy
Physiotherapist came. Jason says he will walk later.

5 p.m.
Still no walking. Mom went back to the hotel. I ask him to go for a walk, but he gets mad at me. I want to push him a little. But I'm scared too. I know he's in pain. But I know he has to get up.

6:45

Dr. S comes in. Asks about Jason. He doesn't want to wake him. But he's been sleeping for an hour or so. I tell him to go ahead. So he takes Jason's hand and tells him he's doing good. He reminds him that he needs to get up and walk. Jason's pretty out of it so I'm not sure if he will remember or listen.

8:30 a.m.

So you didn't get up and walk last night. Today I will force you for your own good.

Not much happened last night. Very up and down. But I think we might have slept a little more. About 3 am he felt very very sick. But didn't throw up. He noticed that one of the night aides increased his food flow, and that made him feel nauseous. We stopped the food altogether around 5 or 6 am. Besides a few readjustments, a few coughs, and some pain and nausea medication it was ok. Very choppy sleep but sleep none the less.

Jason's pretty swollen this morning. He can barely open his eyes. He's in a bit of pain but it seems like the switch to oxy is kind of helping. The goal today is to get him up and moving. Of course you guys know Jason. He's said no last night, but I'm pushing him today. He needs to move so he doesn't get blood clots. I am giving him forty-five minutes from now cause they just gave him some oxy and anti-nausea medicine.

9 a.m.

Jason is feeling nauseous even though he is on Zofran. He had gravel at 7 a.m., so there is nothing else they can give him. I hate when he's on oxy. He just threw his clipboard at me because I told him he had to go for a walk. I said it might be better to get it done and over

161

with now because he just puked do he has nothing left to throw up. He keeps procrastinating. I said twenty minutes. He said forty-five. I agreed on forty-five. Then he started to feel sick. Then he puked. Now he doesn't want to go anywhere I told him he has to. So he's angry. He also thinks he puked last night but he did not. He just felt I'll. the nurses took twenty-five minutes before they answered the call bell, and it wasn't even a nurse. It was the nurse aide Carmen. She's nice but I don't think Jason likes her humor. Our nurse Dianna is gone in break or something. There are only two nurses for the entire ward. I'm frustrated because I can't do anything and neither do they. The one nurse that they have gone in is very dismissive and that makes me mad. She's says she can't give him gravel or anything until 5 p.m. And pretty much just said, oh well. Too bad. Nothing I can do. She didn't even offer to clean him up or anything. I asked for new bandages cause his have puke all over them and she said Dianna would clean it up when she got back. How long will he have to sit in his own filth?

10 a.m. Our nurse Dianna is back. She cleans Jason's bandages up and gives him more medicine. She says by 11 she wants him in the chair. And preferably walking around.

10:45
Resident nurse Franny is on the unit instead of Dr. S. She was here last time. She didn't do this surgery, but helped a see done questions about the yellow patch on his face. It's a smaller skin graft. Not what they call a flap. He's still sleeping. He slept through her while visit. But she says things are looking good. The swelling goes up before it goes down.

11:20.
I force you to walk around. I'm mean like that. You went 1/2 way. I know it's hard. Better than nothing for sure. The nurse and I give

you a sponge bath. The nurse says I'm a good wife. Made me feel nice. We sat you in the chair for a bit.

2:30
I went back to the hotel to take a shower and rest a bit. My mom stayed at the hospital. I came back at 5 pm. Mom said you pooped right after I left. And you were pooping when I came back. She said you sat in your chair for a good hour. And watched 2 game of thrones without me. 6 pm mom went home to red deer. I watch 1/2 of an episode of game of thrones. Then the stupid thing shut down. Pissed me right off.

7:15.
Jason is having trouble breathing. I cleaned out the inner cannula for him. He says it's not helping. He has been waiting for respiratory therapy since 4 pm. The in-call nurse gave us a hard time for asking to use the suction. I said listen. He hasn't used it. He thinks it will help do it. So she did. It didn't help. Then she told us about how the body needs nutrition to heal etc.. Still waiting on respiratory.
She said he would be in in five minutes. That was half an hour ago. You wrote you are dying. I said no. You said this isn't living...

7:30
Our night nurse came to do vitals and check on him. She said respiratory nurse got called away. But we would be first when he did his rounds. I'm pretty sure Jason has an infection on his new neck skin. I point it out to the nurse. She will have the doctor look at it tomorrow. They haven't been as good with the cleaning of his incisions and putting the polymers on it this time. Hopefully they change his bandages soon. They are looking dirty. Jason and I decided a lit if his nausea is coming from the oxy. We are going to see if Tylenol will work for the times between the pain medicine ... It's worth a shot.

Hopefully he can get this nausea under control so he can start to eat and get more energy to walk around. He wrote he's thirsty.

8 pm.

Respiratory nurse comes to check on him. Cleans everything up and Instills him with water. Still doesn't help. His oxygen levels and good, but he has decreased air flow coming out of his trachea. They are going to order medicine to help him breath for now. He thinks Jason is having trouble breathing because of all the swelling. He is very swollen and that makes it hard for him right now. You wrote that I was a great nurse. A pain in the ass, but a great nurse. After the respiratory guy sprayed you with water and you couldn't catch your breath you wrote you can do much more of this. The respiratory guy says you can. It's got to get worse before it will get better. You wrote you are still thirsty.

He's afraid of stopping breathing. I would be too but the respiratory nurse assures him he will be ok. Jason wrote he doesn't remember this part of it last time. Or it being this hard.

Sunday, July 13

The night was OK. Jason was up a lot of the night. Very restless. He leg has been giving him some grief, but he now has decided not to use oxy because it makes him nauseous. He hasn't had oxy for a day now. Just extra strength Tylenol and Gravel. He says his pain is at a five, except for when I touch the nose tube. Then it's at a ten. It's so, so hard not to touch that fucking stupid nose tube. Today he punched/grabbed me because as I was unhooking his oxygen it came loose sudden and I hit his nose tube kind of hard. I didn't mean to but holy shit he was mad. On another note, I had him sit in the chair for an hour, then he walked, but not as far as yesterday. And yesterday wasn't far. He was out of breath. He has a weird bump on his lower back that kind of looks like fluid. But it's hard not squishy like fluid. The on call doctor says his neck incision doesn't look infected but just keep an eye on it. I also noticed his Iv was not working cause his arm got all swollen and big. They are going to have him on day round nausea medicine, and so far it's seeming to help. Today, I'm an going to see if we can have Gravel only at night because it helps him sleep. Everything else is good. He's not as swollen today, which is good. Just got to get him up for a walk again later today. :)

6 p.m.
My mom is getting ready to leave. She and Jason walked two times! Awesome. Since his IV came out, he's seriously doing amazing. So if course he thinks it's his IV, lol. Whatever works. He's on a low dose of tramacet. It's stronger than extra strength Tylenol, but less strong than Oxy. So his nausea has significantly decreased since he went off Oxy. Of course they want to put the stupid Iv back in just in case something happens to his breathing. But hopefully they can wait for a while. The Tramacet and Tylenol are keeping his pain managed, which is awesome cause that means when he leaves he won't have to wean off the oxy. I really don't like it when he's on the oxy. His back is still sore and of course his leg is very sore. And he gets pressure headaches, but he's increased his food to fifty-five, and we will see how that goes. Right now he is not even getting enough food to sustain his weight. But it's not good to feed fast and have him vomit everything up. So slow and steady. He's really thirsty since no Iv. But gets water flushes from his nose tube. He was in really good spirits this afternoon. And was joking and laughing when I gave him his present (a fox that sings what does the fox say) he was chatting with my mom and going for walks. All in all the best day do far. Let's keep this going lol.
(three days ago, Oxy story)
He looked at mom, and she had a small robot crawling on her face
Then he looked at me and I had the small snake from Beetlejuice crawling in my eye ...

8:30 p.m.
Jason has to get a new IV. Fred is doing it On His hand. Ouch. Mike and his wife just left. Good visit. They make Jason laugh. And they both said how awesome he looks and is doing. Mike goes for chemo tomorrow. Hopefully it goes well. They are a super nice couple. I really like them and their company.

9:30 p.m.
Best day bust. I went downstairs to get supper. He vomited when the night nurse decided to turn his feeding tube up to fifty-five cc an hour; he turned it down to forty-five, and that was still up by 10cc an hour but it's frustrating because Dianna said they were going to leave it for twelve hours because he's been so nauseous. Either she didn't write that down in the chart or the night guy didn't read the chart, but that makes me so angry because it puts him back a few steps now. The rest of the night was ok.

Monday July, 14
Went for a walk. Sat in chair. No pain medicine except extra strength Tylenol. Stayed awake most if the day; having problems breathing again, got the nurse to give a few puffs of the inhaler. No vomiting. Went for another walk. My dad came to visit. Watched a few movies on the laptop. Got dad To bring up game of thrones. He offered to get me supper. I said ok. He drove all over town looking for Greek Food for me. Couldn't find one. Got Gravel. Went to bed at 12 a.m, Jason says his breathing is still tight. Up at 2 am readjusting and peeing. Around 4 am he gets some more puffs even though he's sleeping. 5:30 the night nurse tells us he's going to give Jason pain medicine because they are taking down the dressings today.

Tuesday, July 15, 6:15 am (day 7)

Today they took Jason's leg dressings down. It was a bit painful at the top where the skin grafts are. The gauze stuck to the cut and pulled to take off. There is a large skin flap on the lower leg. I thought the skin flaps came from the thigh only. Jason has lots of staples to keep him closed right now. Waiting for doctor to come in. 6:45, doctor comes. Says everything is looking good. Going to keep trachea in and staples in leg. Keep walking, etc.

Dr. S came by today too. He says you need to walk every four hours today and every two hours tomorrow.

You only did one set of exercises today. But you walked two and a half times.

Wednesday, July 16

2 a.m. You. Vomited. You have been feeling sick for an hour or more. You had Gravol and we stopped the tube feed. Sigh.

The rest of Wednesday was good. Steven Dalton came to and brought breakfast at around 10:30 a.m.

You got a side neck drain, the left one, taken out. Steven stayed till 3 p.m., when Anton came here and visited. Anton stayed till almost six.

Mom came at six and visited till eleven. You walked five times. And sat up in the chair a bit.

Thursday, July 17

Opened up leg dressings and took a look. They said they could take out every second staple except where the graft was on the lower leg. Took out both dopplers in your neck. And downsized your trach tube to a 4. If you can breathe through it and the swelling goes down more, they can cap it and get that stupid trach out. The respiratory tried to plug your tube and get you to say hi. But you are blowing air around the tube because your upper airways are so swollen right now.

Not a bad afternoon or night. A little breathless so didn't want to walk as much. But still walked a bit. Visited with my mom and watched some shows. Looks like you are finally starting the uphill climb!! Yay you.

Friday, July 18

Night was OK. Every four hours someone wakes us up.

6 a.m. Doctor wakes us up to see how we are. Thinks things are going well. Getting the last neck drain tube out.

Oh no. Your nose tube is all plugged. Shit, shit, shit. If they can't get it unplugged, you need to go for surgery to get a new one. Finally used some enzymes and got it unplugged. Got all looked at and went for a walk. I ate free pancake breakfast. You fed yourself a box of food, then vomited everywhere. We noticed that your nose tube was in the wrong place. Also after vomiting you need suction but something is stuck in the airways. So now they want to send you for a scope and an X-ray also. 2 steps forward. :(one back. The nurses think you are more swollen than yesterday.

Saturday, July 19

Plugged the trachea tube. Said if you can breathe through that you can get it out on Monday. At night you found it very hard to breathe. Took it out.

Sunday July 20.

You were quite swollen again. Doctors say in Monday they will take trach out and on Tuesday they will take drain in leg out and get you to start eating foods.

Well, the afternoon was good. Sister and mom were here. We painted rocks. And I made a paper mâché butterfly. Then around four, auntie Della and Jim came to visit. We had supper then they left. After they left you had a meltdown.

I asked if you were ready for your walk, and if you had done your exercises. Well, that was it. You told me that the swelling wasn't going down. And there was no point in walking. I reminded you the doctors said you should walk. You said you weren't walking so move the computer to you so you can watch it. I said sure. Right after you walk. You had a fit and threw the pen at me and told me to leave. So I gave you the computer and I left. You said you talked to the nurse and she said your white chin will always be like that. I say let's listen to the doctor. He said it will go down, so it will. It just takes time. You are very frustrated tonight. With everything. Your leg hurts, you can form speech well yet (day 2 of plugging the trach.) but you are frustrated. You were very rude to the respiratory nurse tonight. You told her you wanted the trach plug off and she said to try laying down with it I'm first. Then you guys argued for a bit. Essentially, she says that it takes time. You are only 11 days out if surgery. I don't like it when you ask the nurses if they have had a bone taken out or if they are missing a tongue. It's like a pity party for you. It's ok to feel frustrated but you don't have to be nasty about it. No one close to you knows what you are going through. The nurses have seen a lot though. They do have a good idea of what is going on and why they do things. But every person is different and heals different. No one can feel how you feel. But please remember. There are people who are way worse off then you. At least you get to see you daughter and son grow up. And least you can walk you little girl down the aisle. At least you can hear them call you daddy. You have your hands. You can write to us or your kids. Your family doesn't care how you look. I know it's hard but let's try to put a positive spin on this. I am here if you need to vent, or cry or scream. But I don't like it when you throw things at me. It feels like an attack on me. And I'm trying my very best here. You don't know what it feels like to be me. To see your husband suffering and upset and angry and to be able to do absolutely not one single thing to help. I feel useless. I feel like I don't even need to be here because you are tired of me asking you to go on walks and to eat and to exercise. Fuck I hate asking you to do it. But it seems like if I don't remind you, you don't do it. And the only one suffering is you. But I don't want you to suffer. That's the issue. So understand that the doctors have seen this 190x before. They have seen people just like you. They have seen people who don't get up and don't get better and they have seen people that do get up and get better. They are telling you what works. For yourself.

Monday July 21

So I told on you. Told the doctors that you didn't think the swelling in your neck would ever go down. And that you were angry that the tongue would never lift up. They said the swelling would go down. You need to walk. After they left you fed yourself and I asked if you wanted to walk. You said no. A social worker came. We went to a head and neck cancer meeting. I liked it. You said it was pointless. You did some work. Sister came to visit. You only had two walks all day. A little sad that you are not listening to doctors.

Tuesday, July 22

Night was very long. Jason was up every 1/2 hour. But on a good note, he did sleep with the trach plugged all night. But I think he was afraid he would choke or something. They say that he gets his leg drains out today. One less thing to carry around when walking. He needs to walk more. He only walked 3x all of yesterday and the doctors want him to walk every 2 hours. Hopefully he will do more today. Telling him to walk doesn't do anything but make him upset, so don't bother.

He is also getting the stitches in his chin incision out today. He still has quite a bit of swelling although the doctors are saying it's going down, it's not going down fast enough for Jason. Every day seems to get a bit better. We both like the visits and the pictures and videos of the kids do keep sending them!

He got the zero-form off and every 2nd stitch from his leg out. We met with the physio guy and he taught Jason's a few tricks when he is walking. So walking is going better today. He's walked more today than ever before.

July 23.
Rough night again. Nights are bad. He took cap off trach at 2 am. That means he can't get the trach tube out for another few days. He's swollen up a lot again today. He's coughing a lot today again. The mean respiratory nurse was in again today and says there is no real reason for him to not be plugged. He needs to stop unplugging his trach or he will have it in for a lot longer. He needs to practice swallowing better. And to walk more, so that the swelling goes down. So pretty much the same thing they tell us every day. He's now had his trach in for fifteen days. They usually take it out on Day 6. He's having a tough time with the trach because it irritates his esophagus because it's not sitting right. He did really well walking yesterday. Hopefully he's not too sore and we can keep that going today.

July 24
They took out the trach because we asked for it out. He's doing better walking. The night was hard because he kept choking on his phlegm. But he's happy because the trach is out. The speech lady

came in to help with his swallowing. She told us that he'd had a total glossectomy. We did not know that. Makes swallowing very hard. Very upsetting to hear. They told us that he would never eat or talk well again. He will be in a liquid for the rest of his life. He practiced with swallowing water and the speech lady was very happy with that. He asked for a weekend pass. He got it.

July 25

Let's blow this Popsicle stand. Jason wants out now. So we get ready to go. The day nurse is very nice. She gets all his meds and stuff ready.

CHAPTER 31

Adapting To My New Reality

Reading up to this point, I hope I have confirmed that I was basically a normal guy living a normal life—and it felt as though it was all coming to an end, but un sure when that end may be. Things were not going like they hoped though I did make it through the very long recovery stage since the removal of the bottom half of my face, I was devastated when (through the careless unforgiving eyes from one of the top surgeons in the Country) while using a voice that you would use to order a hamburger. I was given the news I was telling me that I was going to die within about three months. I was not at all expecting that as it came out of the blue and hit me like the front end collision in a car accident. During the time it took processing the new reality that I faced , I looked back on my life and I had a few regrets, some of which I have already written about.

Though I was very scared to die, I was confident that I had lived my life well. I had a great childhood with loving parents, and I had a part in creating an amazing family, whom I love so dearly. I worried about who my wife would have to go out with on dates and if they would treat her like a lady, I worried who would be my kids role model when it came to a more masculine role model, I worried the impact and hurt my kids would feel the day of and after my funeral, I worried about being forgotten forever. And I worried so much that I hurt , that my kids would remember me distant memory that you remember more so from the stories people tell of you and less memories that we shared together. But, I knew I had a strong wife and two great kids, and I knew deep down that, if I must die, it would be OK.

Here's what cancer did to me , I had gone from being a man that society would label as totally normal, to being labeled as disabled by exact definition of the word. . I had to re-learn to walk, talk/ communicate, eat, and breathe, all while continuing to financially support my family, and I had to relearn what would work best for me in approaching this new reality. I also had to prove to myself that my mind was still fully functioning and working normally. Because I couldn't physically use my voice anymore, I had to go back to using primitive means of communicating. Like I was back to being a toddler, using drawings and throat noises to get things I needed. With these limitations, I needed to figure out a way to become just as successful as I had been.

So during my uphill battle with cancer, while doing whatever it took to keep my ass alive, I now thought of myself as a freak, which is not the way to live life, but I was so angry that I couldn't do any- thing about it. You see, my looks were always so important to me and, to be honest, they still are. Now my new face is permanently fucked up and I hate it. I am reminded of this every time I speak, eat, drink, or look in a mirror. Especially when I talk I am reminded, because I have to wipe the drool from my mouth. It's really hard to have confidence in yourself when you must constantly wipe your mouth like you would a two-month-old baby. The only thing that didn't change about me through this was the way my brain worked.

Because my brain works the same as it always has, I hated it when people would look in disgust at my face when I walked by—not because they were trying to be rude, but because that's their instinctive reaction to something that is out of place. And my face sure isn't proportionally correct anymore. Later on during my rehabilitation, my physiotherapist, who had not read my file in its entirety and didn't know that my lower jaw had been reconstructed, literally pushed my jaw out of its socket while trying to stretch out my neck from the radiation fibrosis. So now my jaw permanently opens crooked as well. Too bad she didn't have more training.

Though I hate how I look, it's a constant reminder that I am in this battle every minute of every waking hour of my life. Still, I've never truly felt sorry for myself. You see, life as I knew it was not even close to the same; everything in my day to day life had to change. I went from being a very well-off and successful businessman to being broke, in what literally felt like a moment. I went from being able to speak clearly to not at all, from eating and chewing food with my mouth to blending it and injecting it into my stomach through a feeding tube. Hell, I went from breathing normally to breathing out of a fucking trachea. I had been a normal fucking guy and was forced to be a man who dribbles coffee down the front of his shirt. And I felt as though I had to act like this was all normal, because this very quickly became my new reality. Which was coming to a very quick end. Oddly enough this was a bit of a saving grace when it came to my expiration date, because I was not very ok with myself as a person anymore.

CHAPTER 32

Trying To Hold It Together

My suggestion for anyone that needs to keep their sanity while stuck in a hospital bed, regardless of the diagnosis, is to focus on something else, like a project, and set some goals for yourself. My own personal goals were not what I would recommend to others, as they could get you in trouble or make you feel like a total ass (as mine did with some family members). However, I do suggest you focus on something other than this stupid disease. Having a task to complete made it so I couldn't be in my head all day, every day, feeling sorry for myself. This, I truly believe, was the key to having a positive attitude, and I know for certain that it played a major part in my cancer battle.

In my own personal situation, I was receiving a consistent flow of bad news—so much that it became mind-blowingly devastating to me and us. My worst nightmares were becoming a reality. At first, it wasn't so bad, as I felt like I could see a light at the end of the tunnel because the doctors kept presenting me with solutions—like surgeries, and then chemo and radiation—but as that light kept fading, I had to cling to anything I could to help me stay positive. Maybe that's the key to beating cancer, or maybe not, but for me it was the only way to keep hope alive. It felt as though my nightmares were coming to life.

The first of the bad news was getting the diagnosis of cancer. When I eventually received the diagnosis, it was already in Stage 4, so my odds weren't looking too bad. For me, hearing the news wasn't as bad as I thought it would be; it was more of an inconvenience. I did get emotional and cried to my boss while I told him, but that was more because I had to quit my job because of the cancer and not so much because I was scared for my life. In the position I was in as a corporate HR/safety rep, I couldn't perform the duties of the job because I probably would never talk again. Thankfully, he didn't accept my resignation. His response was, "Let's just do what we always do, and we will re-assess the situation as things arise; no need to worry even before you know the hurdle. But for now, let's just keep it to ourselves."

The doctors told me they had to act fast and that they were going to perform a major invasive surgery, taking half my tongue, and then they hit me with huge doses of chemo and radiation. The doctors' exact words were, "You're going to get very sick before you can get better." I was told the struggle in life would be harder but living a life without half a tongue would be manageable.

Second: After that surgery, I was told everything had gone as well as planned and we started chemo and radiation. This was a really low point during this entire journey, and I really needed something positive in my life. The chemo and radiation were honestly fucking brutal—but more so the radiation, which I found surprising. From what I'd read on the internet, I figured the chemo would be bad. But it was nothing when you compare it to the final half of the remaining rounds of radiation. And that's excluding the feeling you get every time they strap you to that platform and place the meshed mask on your face. These masks are specifically made to form to every curvature and dimension of your face, and they clip you down to the platform so you are physically not able to move your head even a millimetre. It's exactly how I always imagined a psychiatric patient would be restrained prior to shock therapy its really a whole new level of scariness. The treatments were typically a forty-five-minute ordeal, from what I recall being told. Thinking back, I can't remember, but that's probably because I spent the years since then blocking the sensation of how that felt out of my brain. Knowing I had to do this again the next day and ay after that on a continual basis made me want to just die. The radiation sucked the life out of me so fast that I noticed the change in my appearance every day when I looked in the mirror. Three rounds of chemo and thirty-three of radiation is not something the human body was supposed to be exposed to.

Third: The cancer came back, and with a vengeance, and I had to get put back into the hospital. It was at this point that they decided to remove my entire tongue and I was told I would never be able to talk again. Imagine never being able to talk to your kids again or tell your wife you love her? I know there are other means of communicating, like hand gestures or writing things down, but it's just not the same. With the return of the cancer, I was sure I was going to lose my job, which meant I knew I would be living without a consistent income to support my family. But again, after talking to my boss, the VP said he would keep me on as I was doing really well with my reports and reaching my deadlines.

Fourth: they removed my entire tongue, replaced three quarters of my lower jaw with my left leg bone, and then pieced me back together. Most of the skin, muscle, and bone they removed came from the left side of my body and was placed somewhere else. The hospital sheets were constantly soaked with my blood, body fluids, and puss. I spent a very long time in recovery. I thought that this was the end of my life and that my fight was over, not realizing that it was just the beginning and that the real battle had yet to start.

Fifth: I'm not sure how long I was out of the hospital for, but one day my wife had to rush me to the emergency department. The cancer (due to swelling) was somehow blocking my airway, and I was literally suffocating to death. At that time, I was rushed into surgery, where they installed a new trachea (again) so I could breathe. I didn't know it at the time, but this was my new reality. I was going to have this trachea for the rest of my life. You know the commercial where the person smokes through the hole in their throat? Yeah, that was how my life would be now. Not only could I not talk or eat, but now I had to breathe through a hole in my neck for the rest of my life. That had to be the worst of it … or so I thought.

Sixth: The doctor explained to me why the cancer had spread and the reason for all the swelling and the sores on my face. They said the cancer was like those mushrooms that are full of dust-like spores, the kind that poof up like an explosion when you disturb them in any way. Knowing what had happened, they did that second major surgery, which was basically a rescue mission to correct something that had previously gone terribly, terribly wrong. I'm sure a doctor can explain this better, but this is how it was explained to me. At that point I was told, "You have three months left and there is nothing I can do about it. You need to come to terms with this as fast as you can so you can enjoy your final days." I told my boss this right away and he brought this news to the board of trustees. Who all agreed to keep me employed until my final living day … given that the prognosis was only three months to live.

CHAPTER 33

Another Uphill Battle Begins

In October 2014, I was given the news that I only had three months left to live. I did everything in my power to ensure that, though I was dying, I would be able to continue to live as normally as I did before, because I didn't want to miss out on one more thing in my in life.

For those of you who don't know us personally, my wife and I create annually an amazing Halloween-night experience for the kids in our neighborhood. It's one of the top-five most important days of the year to us. We have a different theme each time, so it's a new experience for every kid and parent every year. We always have a popcorn maker and a huge turkey deep fryer pot full of hot chocolate, which I proudly am always in charge of. But even though all of my heart was still in it, I was not able to muster the energy to even go outside on this particular Halloween. I could hear the screams and laughter coming from the window of my bedroom, but I didn't have the strength to go outside and see it, let alone participate. But fortunately, it still went on as planned with my good friends, who dressed up as zombies that year. My sister even came for this particular Halloween to make it even more kick-ass. At home in Vancouver, she is in charge of the set designs for some of the biggest motion pictures that are filmed there. Worked on movies like the first *Deadpool*

180

(that's right, my sister is super bad-ass!), *Fifty Shades of Grey, Magic Mike, Big Eyes* by Tim Burton, *Van Helsing,* and many more. She was so good that she was specifically requested to set up the large musical performances for Magic Mike in London and Germany.

So my sister and my brother-in-law (who's also in the set-designing business) came to visit and took charge of creating the best Walking Dead themed Halloween house you could ever imagine! The pictures don't even do it justice. From that year on, she has done everything in her power to make sure she is available to help me out with decorating our house for all the kids in our neighborhood. The trick or treaters that actually make it past the zombies and get to the front door get juice or a pop can with a glow stick, and of course a package of dental floss and a toothbrush (the perks of living with a dental hygienist, lol). We also give out a prize for the cutest and scariest costume, and, of course, the kids and adults can also have popcorn and hot chocolate.

We had a lot of actors in my circle of friends—hell, even my best friend, Steve, flies from Vancouver every year to be a part of the fun.

Prior to October, I had these open sores on the sides of my cheeks, and by this point, my face was blown up like a balloon and I had lost so much weight I resembled a skeleton and weighed only 101 pounds. I do have one picture of me from then, but I decided against adding it to the book because I still can't bear to look at myself like that. These open sores had turned into quarter-sized open wounds. These open wounds, which were on both cheeks, oozed puss and blood and kept growing. It was nasty, and I also had to check myself into the hospital because I couldn't breathe. The swelling was so bad that it was three-quarters of the way blocking my airway, so the doctor had to insert another trachea. I didn't know at the time, but that was to be a permanent thing for the rest of my life.

Also at this point, the incisions on the sides of my neck started to open up like my cheeks did—open pits filled with puss and dead skin that was beige in color and would come off in small pieces like wet plaster. And don't even get me started on the smell of the decaying flesh, which was unescapable due to the fact that my cheeks were literally rotting off me.

This time when I was re-diagnosed with this cancer, it had rapidly spread all through my body. It was found in the back of my skull, in my lungs, armpits, and of course on my neck and face. By this time, it was peppered all over my body. It was in my bloodstream and spreading like wildfire. I was then told I was in Stage 4 and terminal. Now I am making up these numbers, as I don't have the slightest clue how they calculate the margins, but I will use my made-up numbers to help explain what was explained to me. Let's say you have a five-by-five-centimeter infected cancerous area. They will cut out about one-and-a-half times the infected area—so in this case, their margins would be seven-and-a-half centimeters squared, around the center of the infected area. If I had known this before the first surgery, I would have told them to take the whole tongue the first time around, long before they ever told me they were going to cut it as close as possible to try and save my tongue. I struggled to talk after they removed the first part of my tongue, and I wouldn't be doing much talking if I was dead anyway. To be honest, knowing how sick I would get, I would have wanted the doctors to remove it all in the first place. I wish I could go back in time and tell the doctor to remove it all and not take the risk in trying to save some of my tongue just to stroke his ego to attempt to prove how great he was. I don't feel like it's ethical or fair to his patients that he risk their lives all while experimenting with risky procedures not knowing the outcome. If he had just cut a wider chunk out of my tongue, it's possible the cancer may not have spread everywhere and at such a rapid rate. Maybe it would have spread slowly over time, but that's just it,

I would have had more time with my family. If he had known that the cancer was larger than what was showing up in the last CT scan and that he may not be able to get all of it, and if he didn't it would probably spread at a rapid speed and kill me, I would have had some options. I would have chosen to be way more aggressive and take all of my tongue! But he didn't explain that to me or offer me any other options. He assured me that he would, without a doubt, be able to remove all of the cancer. *He fucking promised me that.* But because of his error and lack of care, he cut into the cancer, and that is what caused it to spread so rapidly!!

With no emotion or compassion in his voice, he said, "I give you maybe about three months to live, so just go home and face what's to come." And then he handed me a prescription for about a million Oxycodone pills and sent me on my way. We went from *I promise I will remove your cancer* to *Don't waste my time and go home and die.*

I am editing this for a fourth time and removing some of the evil comments I put in here, as I don't want to be perceived as a complete asshole. But when the one guy I was told I could trust says he will not give up on me and then just flicks me away like the butt end of a cigarette without showing one single ounce of remorse, then obviously I have some words for him about his unprofessional and unethical behavior. As well, his skills aside, I really feel he is a heartless prick who's just in it for the money. ← DR's need to be more Careful + not make promises

That being said, I do want him to know that he really can do some amazing work. After my first surgery, you couldn't tell that I had literally been sliced from ear to ear across my throat. But the moment he decided that I was a lost cause, he didn't care about his workmanship and wrote me off without giving me any kind of hope. I really feel that he could have looked into other options and offered me other choices when the cancer came back the second time and he definitely could have done a better job and made me look more normal, especially knowing first hand how capable he actually was.

This is just how I perceive it; maybe he saw it differently. But at the end of the day, I know what I saw, and I saw this doctor looking at me as if I were a walking corpse that he wanted out of his office, as I was taking up space and wasting his time.

You know, Doctor, I hope that someday this happens to you. Not the cancer stuff, because I don't wish for anyone to have to go through what I did, not even Malady, but I hope one day you experience the same treatment that you gave me from a doctor or lawyer who delivers bad news and doesn't show one lick of empathy and just wants you out of his office. I don't wish the doctor any ill will, but maybe he could hire a shitty divorce lawyer, or maybe he could get a ticket for not yielding to oncoming traffic from an arrogant police officer, like what happened to me with the old lady, so that he can experience what it feels like to be treated like shit by a person of authority.

What my doctor didn't know was that my closest family and friends were never going to give up on me, no matter what the circumstances. Though my group was small, they were very reliable and resourceful in researching everything possible to find a way to help me survive this. The help, research and time that all my family and friends gave me was more than I knew at the time, but appreciate so much now. For me personally, my doctor's actions toward me and my case forced me to give up on myself. But my real family and friends stood beside me every step of the way and inspired me to keep going. These are the only people I want in my life, and I know without a shadow of a doubt that if they had to, they would carry my faintest-of-breath body across the finish line to win this uphill battle. And that's exactly what they did.

My family found ways to move mountains and leap entire oceans to make whatever they needed to make happen, happen, no matter the obstacles they faced. I need you all to know that I love you with all my heart!

184

My wife was incredibly determined and spent many hours researching options for immunotherapy in Arizona and planning on doing whatever it took to get me there. My sister had me on this regimen of acids and or bases that would somehow comingle or neutralize the pH in my blood that caused cancer. My wife also put me on a phoenix tear cannabis solution that I had to take every night to assist in fighting off the cancer. I was forced into pathologists' offices and foot-detoxing places. The only thing they didn't try was an exorcism, which I was actually thinking of adding to the itinerary at my funeral ceremony just to fuck with people. They were researching every avenue to give me the best fighting chance.

Then, through persistent questioning and not accepting what was said to be my fate, my wife discovered a trial for a drug called nivolumab for head and neck cancers, in Vancouver. My family did whatever they had to do to get me on the trial.

It was around the time I started the immunotherapy that I started the phoenix tear drops,. I kept taking the tears every day as well as the trial schedule. Every night like clockwork, I was high as a kite before I went to bed. You know how it's fun to get drunk once in a while, but not two night in a row? Well, I had to get stoned. But not just once in the week. I had to do this every single day for three months, regardless of whether I wanted to get high or not. I hated it so much. I wasn't myself at all. But hell, it was only three months, which was doable—or so I thought, as I craved McDonald's fries and burnt toast.

Soon after I started the tears and immunotherapy, a had a bit more strength, not that I was strong but within two months, I was able to walk down the stairs again without assistance, and my body seemed to stop getting worse which was a relief, which happened shortly after I had fully given up on myself. Now imagine if my doctor had said, "Well, we tried cutting it out and it didn't work, so maybe we should try experimental trials before we cut out your whole tongue and completely fuck up your life" instead of going in for that second surgery and saying just take it all out. If we knew there was immunotherapy, be it experimental or proven, like in Arizona, we would have made an executive decision. But he told us that our only option was to remove the whole tongue and we believed him, because we were told we could trust him. Knowing how difficult the recovery was the first time, the last thing I wanted to do was re-live that experience again. I would have tried anything else.

I learned through this experience that surgery isn't always the only answer. Sometimes science can help too. And if my old surgeon knew more than just how to cut, maybe he would have done more research and looked at other options and said, "I think this needs a different approach." Maybe I would be living a normal life now, without the permanent trachea, stomach tube, or constant drool dripping off my lip. I would still have half a tongue that would allow me to eat, drink, and talk. Now for the rest of my life I can't kiss my wife properly without worrying that some drool might get on her lips. This is my life now.

The kicker was that my mind worked amazingly, almost to the point that issues became too easy to problem solve. My mind was sharp as a razor, but my body was diseased and crippled. Getting my work done was simple, but the hardest thing for me was putting the laptop down, getting out of bed, and taking a shower. Some days, that was a six-hour ordeal; on others, it just wasn't something I could do. Many times, my wife would find me curled up in the fetal position on the shower floor, trying to build up enough energy to not only endure the feeling of intense cold when I opened the shower door, but to also be able to dry myself off. Taking a shower was a goal that I reached for each and every day. It was tough, but I was managing.

And then I got kicked again.

CHAPTER 34

Humiliated At Home

Things seemed to be going quite smoothly in my work life at this time. I was still doing all my program updating and computer work from the hospital bed or home bed. I just emailed or texted the people I needed to talk to, which actually was so much easier because I could confirm the dates and times and had evidence of the exact wording in every conversation. So, in some respects, I was doing even more efficient work, because literally everything was now fully accounted for and documented. Nothing was getting lost in translation in what used to be actual verbal conversations. But then Mr. Red was fired because of the greedy corporate assholes who didn't want to have to pay him his well-earned bonus. And with him out of the picture (the only office person who was looking out for me and my family), all they had to do was wait a bit to let the smoke clear and then get rid of the guy with cancer.

I was fired from the company because I had cancer. (I don't understand how the key people who actually knew how much time, blood, sweat, and tears I had put into that company would be on board with this.) So now I was just fucking mad at the world—I was so incredibly angry all the time. My boss had decided to come over to my house completely unannounced, except for the call they placed to say they were two minutes away and stopping by so we could talk. They showed up un-invited, and I thought it might have been a friendly visit to check up on the condition of their employee and say how good of a job I was doing. But they sat down with me at my kitchen table and had the nerve to fire me right there in my kitchen, all while my daughter was ten feet away playing while listening to these people tell me how I was not good enough for them anymore. Would that change the way she saw me as her father? Did they just make my daughter hear that her tough, strong dad was actually a loser who wasn't good enough? Seriously, why not call me into head office and fire me there? Or over the phone, or by email, or hell, even with a text? But how could they—and how dare they— do it in my fucking home when my kid was home? The disrespectful pricks. How the hell did they get to where they are with these morals? Every time I look at my dining room table, I am reminded of being fired in front of my daughter there. They took comfort and security away from me in the place I should always feel the safest. They are either that unethical or really that fucking stupid. Either way, I need them to know how inappropriate that was and that you both are actually bad people! Firing me in my home in front of my daughter crushed my soul. You made me lose all confidence, any dignity I had was de-masculinized. Though I thought it was a possibility, I couldn't actually believe my head office would abandon their employees in their greatest time of need. The problem when these types of people, the type without a moral compass, make it into these office positions is that they backstab their way to the top. I am an exception because not only did I work my ass off to get to where I was before they fired me, but because I mainly lucked out by answering a phone at the right time.

Un like them, I didn't need to stab anyone in the back to rise the ladder; the ony thing I did was get payback for what that other manager did to me and my family by putting our finacial security at risk. It took a while, but I did get you back, you selfless prick. Though I am glad you landed on your feet and got a job where you would have more time at home and would get paid a lot more than before. In fact, you were able to buy that house on the lake because of this. But I did have to make you lose your job, as I couldn't trust you in that kind of position. Just know that we are now even. Oh, also, when they called about a reference on you, I did tell them all the good things about you, as we did have fun and worked well together for years and years, but I couldn't go on with a clear conscience knowing you gladly fucked me over and jeopardized my family's income just to dodge getting caught in a lie you were guilty of.

I tried not to show my anger that often (sorry, hon, that you always saw the worst), but after that situation, I couldn't help it. Inside, I was raging like a pissed-off bull that saw people for what they were: selfish. Because of the effects of cancer, it felt like someone literally flipped a switch, and I hated everything. I was mad at the world and wanted the world to feel it. How the fucking hell did I get tongue cancer, of all things? And who could I blame? Mom, for one. For over a year, I was mad at her and Dad. (I'm really sorry, but I am on trial here and need to let everyone know the whole story.) I needed a scapegoat, and Mom and Dad (my birth parents) were the ones who made me. So I believed it was their fault for making me a defective body. I was mad at them for a very long time. It was easier to put the blame on my parents than accept that I had somehow done this to myself.

Later on, my sister bought me one of those "23 and Me" family history DNA breakdown things and we found out that the cancer wasn't from my parents, so it had to be an environmental thing. Because I had quit smoking more than ten years before, and the amount of alcohol I drank in a month you could count on one hand, I came to that conclusion because the oil field is where I spent most of my adult life; it had to have been the benzene I was exposed to through all the years, or H2S or something

I was also mad at my father- and mother-in-law. I felt that both families should have been more supportive to me. I don't know what the hell else they could have done for me, but what they *were* doing for me wasn't good enough in my mind. Because of the intense anger I felt, I wasn't thinking logically most of the time. They were always there if I needed them. They watched my kids—hell, they made a schedule for themselves to ensure everything was well taken care of. But I still felt like they needed to do more. I was even mad at my sister. I was mad at the people who would never give up on me. I would yell at them or tell them off on an almost daily basis, just for trying to help.

With no job I knew I was totally fucked. A big part of my anger at this point was directed toward that. Even if I survived the cancer, I had no job. Who was going to interview a guy with no tongue for a job in human resources? My whole life got turned upside down, and I thought, *How the hell are people going to see me now that I feel like I am a burden to society?* I was super proud of the man I had become and the position I held up until this point. I had so many people who respected me, and I appreciated the way people treated me when I was at the top of my game. But after finding out I had cancer and seeing the effects, I was worried people would think I was nothing but a cancer victim or a disabled person and wouldn't even give me the fake respect you get because you are in a higher position than them. I lost all hope when that actually happened.

CHAPTER 35

Science Vs Food

I used to just do what the doctors told me to do, like when they suggested that I use Resource 2.0 (liquid meals) for my breakfast, lunch, and supper every day for life. Well, I tried that, and you know what? Not only did I smell like that "food" (which was basically a mixture of industrial chemicals) all the time, but it was actually making me less and less healthy. This liquid slurry never had to be refrigerated and had the expiry date of paint. Because that was the only food that was in my body, when I sweated, the smell of vanilla (which was used to mask the smell and taste of this chemical concoction) would come out of every sweat gland on my body. My health was diminishing—and fast. Same with my motivation to stay alive. But when my wife finally decided to quit giving me what the doctor insisted I eat and started to blend me up real food, like lasagna or a stew and injected it into my stomach tube, I was a totally different person within days. Granted, I was still mad at the world, but now I was starting to get my strength back, which made me feel like I might be able to finally fight back.

From that time forward, we decided that I would only eat normal, real food. When I say *real* food, I mean the same food that my family ate, from steak and potatoes to salads. Even fast food. My sister of *importance of REAL food.*

course pushed more healthy things, as did my wife, but since the beginning of time I was never a health nut, so I still bitched when they blended up kale, spaghetti squash, or anything out the norm of my usual diet prior to all of this regardless that I would never taste it. For anyone out there that has to eat through a feeding tube, the best blender I found that purées food to the right consistency needed to push it through a feeding tube was the Cuisinart compact portable blending/chopping system. It's about $80 and works like hot damn. Just make sure you use the chopping blade and not the blending blade. I know it's kind of contradictory to what you would think, but it does the best job of everything I have found so far. Just make sure you add enough water and don't overload the blender with food; otherwise, you will end up with paste that takes forever to try to push through. Don't try to blend up wobbly bacon or things with seeds like raspberries or strawberries. Other than that, the sky's the limit.

I did dare one of my best friends to finish a juice-box size of that meal-replacement sludge they gave me, and he told me he felt like shit for two full days after. I don't know why they would ever give that to recovering patients, but I assume it's a money thing. Why give the good stuff to a person who will most likely die anyway? If the doctors/nutritionist encouraged or even just mentioned that I could use real food through the G-tube, we would have done that a long time ago. We just took their word that it was my only option and followed their direction.

In the nutritionist's defense, if they've never actually experienced a feeding tube on their own or known how bad the issue of "food" affected the recovery process, maybe they would have known to try to blend up a steak or hearty meal that could be pushed through an eighth-of-an-inch-diameter hole and been able to give actual suggestions for the recovery process and not just offer a generic solution that they had read in some textbook.

Once I changed my diet and felt more alive—well, as alive as a dying man can feel—I started to focus more on the huge financial burden I had become to my family.

Luckily, I had some of the funds that were raised on my behalf to help out with my medical expenditures, which included travel, medicine, specialty food/vitamins, medical equipment, medical aids, and attachments of all sorts, like extra tracheas, inner cannulas, stomach tubes, and of course cases and cases of Kleenex. So knowing that the finances were limited and would run out at some point, I knew I had to do something to support my family before I was gone or I would leave them in a state of poverty. I didn't want to die, but the longer I lived the more money was spent that they would need.

When I found out I was dying, I had to plan everything in my life to have an expiration date. I felt like I was trapped in a corner with no options, because no one would hire a guy without a tongue, regardless of my experience. And who would hire a guy who was going to die in a few months, not to mention having the rotting flesh on my neck and face that was constantly bleeding and secreting ooze?

Right here during this time in my life I realized there was no hope for me/us, and I would have to do whatever I could with whatever time I had left to secure a future for my family. With nothing to live for, here is where I turned to God. I prayed for the first time in my life. I don't mean how you would pray for something when you're blowing out your birthday candles, but *really* praying, for any sign of a God. I prayed for my literal life, pleading for a second chance and promising that with every part of my heart and soul that I would do it right if I got one. I prayed for any way out of this impossible situation and promised that I would do whatever I needed and pay at any cost.

I felt this once so I get it-

Now I know some people will not believe this, but I saw—well, *felt*—God for the first time then, like really *felt* His presence. It's not like I saw an actual man in front of me, but it was like being on a different level. Things around me almost felt like they were part of an entire working system, and there was a real flow to the world. I would ask God a question, and through the way the wind blew and the color of the sun, I felt like I would get an answer. It's hard to explain something that is more a feeling, but I felt as though my life was operating on a different level. I was amazed with what was happening around me.

Though I am not the religious type that goes to church on Sundays or prays at the side of my bed every night, I do believe that if there is anything after death, now would be the time it would come, as I was feeling almost dead in my mind, body, and soul. I didn't think that a man on death's door could find his spiritual guide, but it happened. Looking back now after more of these encounters, I know exactly what it was, but I initially convinced myself that this unexplainable situation must have been some sort of weird panic attack or a hallucination. I didn't think this could be actually real, so I continued like it never happened.

Though we did have money from a GoFundMe account, we knew it was not going to last forever, so I had to make a plan—and fast. That money was getting burned up pretty quickly on flights, medical supplies, and everyday survival. At this time, things were as scary as they could get for me, and I knew that if I wouldn't give someone like me the time of day if they asked for a job, I couldn't expect someone else to hire me. So I came up with what I felt was my only option!

CHAPTER 36

Knowing When To Pull Pin

While I was in the hospital, we obviously had huge financial worries. While bedridden, I had many thoughts about what, if I was able to move, I was truly willing to do for my family. My first thought was I would rob a bank. I knew I probably wouldn't succeed but knowing my days were numbered , It didn't really matter to me if I died on a bed in a cell, or on a bed in my house. So I figured it was definitely worth a thought or two. How exactly would I do it, and what's the worst that could happen? If I walked into the bank with the intention of robbing it with nothing but a threatening note, the worst thing that could happen would be I got shot and died—great! My family would get some life insurance money. If I died because of cancer, they would get nothing, because I didn't have insurance through my company. And if I lived through the robbery and got arrested, by the time my court/trial date was scheduled, I would be dead anyway. So would it be worth the risk? Hell, yeah! But I felt sure that I could think of something a little more technical/advanced and discreet. So I kept thinking, because the truth of the matter was, due to the lack of strength I had at the time and that it took me a whole day to even prep for a shower, how the fuck could I ever rob a bank and get away with it? There would have to be a pillow laid out on the ground every twenty feet so I could take a nap before I could continue. But I needed to do something for us, because I felt like it was my fault that we had to sell off everything we had worked so hard for all of our adult lives. I was ruining my family's financial stability by the day.

We had to sell off everything we owned, which was stupid because we didn't have any capital in the things we owned because we had bought them on credit and the market had dropped. We owned three houses in total, but as everyone in North America knows, the oilfield is now so unpredictable that the market in Alberta took a shit-kicking. So when we sold the houses, we were fortunate enough to just break even. It killed me that we had to sell the car that my wife bought for me as a birthday present—the sports car of my dreams, a silver 2000 Pontiac Trans Am with black leather interior and T tops. Such a beauty! We also had to sell the half acre of land in Anglemont, which was meant to be our retirement place. We purchased the plot of land next to the one Bambi's parents bought so we could all be together for when we retire and when they need a little more looking after towards the final decades of their lives.

By this point, we had sold everything and things were still getting worse, so we had to do something before we lost the house we were living in. The reason we didn't sell our house yet was because we were going to take such a loss that we would have owed more to the bank than we got for it and would have an extra monthly payment. We even tried to rent it out to see if we could cover the mortgage and us move into a small apartment to save money, but couldn't even get enough to cover the mortgage, let alone the property and city taxes. We were desperate for a solution and could only come up with one solution, but if we were to this we needed to be prepared to take a huge financial hit a few years later on. We knew it was a lose lose situation for us, but at least it would be something that we could plan for in the future and get us through a short period of time to find some sort of solution. To make this happen we needed to try something that was totally foreign to us, which was a rent-to-own situation. Basically, you and the renter come up with a purchase price, and they pay rent for three to five years at a bit of a premium. Then when the term is up, you give a portion of the rent they paid back to them as a secured deposit on the purchase of the house. We knew we were in a sinking ship and that Bambi had no choice but to advance her career so she would be able to make enough money to support the kids after I had passed away. There were dental hygiene schools all over the country that she could have gone to, but the only one at the time with the fastest turnover rate was in Toronto. It was an eighteen-month accelerated program as opposed to the typical three-year program that the other schools offered. We knew we had no choice but for her to do the eighteen-month course, because if I was to die sooner rather than later, it would be so incredibly difficult to go to school full time for three years as well as being a single mom of two young kids. So we agreed to sign the contract for the rent-to-own for our home, sold all our big furniture that we could, and moved across the country to Toronto where we knew no one and didn't have anyone to help support us or me. I knew it was going to be a test of both our wills on both of us as individuals and as a couple. With her at school full time and needing study time, homework time and group project days, I would have to step up as a husband in the role of the home caretaker, and she would have the weight of our entire family's financial future riding on her shoulders. We knew it would be one of the toughest thing our family would have to face but we had no other solutions and were in survival mode.

After driving for four days, we arrived in Toronto and went to our new temporary home that I'd lined up over the internet. It was a very basic two-bedroom apartment for the four of us to live in for the next few years. It wasn't the nicest place, but it was close to a well rated elementary school and was within a 30 min drive for my wife to get to school. We went from a five-bedroom, three-story home to an apartment where the kids shared the master bedroom while Bambi and I took the smaller room. When we moved in, it was close to the middle of summer, and we were housed on the ninth floor of a non-air-conditioned building. It was so incredibly hot, but that was far from our main concern. To our absolute disgust the building was completely infested with hundreds of thousands of cockroaches. The landlord wouldn't even show us the apartment until we signed the lease agreement, knowing full well what we were about to walk into. There were so many around that out of every corner of your eye, there was something constantly skittering by. There were a lot dead on the floor in plain sight because they most likely sprayed the day or two before. Unfortunately because it was an apartment and they were all over, spraying in one suite doesn't destroy the colonies that had taken over the building. When we unloaded the trailer and brought everything inside the apartment, we placed it all in a big pile in the middle of the living room in an attempt to avoid infestation while we looked for a new place that would house the four of us, the two cats, and our dog. It took three days for us to find a different, less infested place, which we lucked into, but the rent was outrageously high, and it was still only a two bedroom. Still, anything was better than what we had. To be honest, it was quite a substantially larger amount than we were paying for our mortgage prior to leaving. But, like I said, it was temporary and a necessity so my family would at least be clean and comfortable while navigating through our new life in the big city.

We moved into the townhouse, which was a huge upgrade from the roach-filled apartment, and got settled in. The kids had mattresses on the floor, as did Bambi and I. It was an incredible sacrifice, but we did what we had to in order to survive. Bambi and the kids went to school, and I did what I could to stay active and sane in a place where I had no family or friends, and no support system whatsoever nearby. While we were in Toronto, I still had to fly once a month to Vancouver for my immunotherapy, which, surprisingly enough, cost about the same as flying from Alberta to Vancouver.

We knew the immunotherapy was doing something right as by this point I had surpassed the 90 days, but we still didn't really know if I was on the road to recovery or if it was just the calm before the storm. The one thing I did know was that I was broke at home in bed and might be getting better but most likely taking a little longer to die like expected.—From my experience when it comes to cases related to this disease, it's always been the latter, so of course I assumed the worst and needed to plan. Now that I figured that bank robbery was out of the question, I needed to come up with a good plan—one that would really work. I was staring at the ceiling one day, and I believed I discovered a flaw in the building design. Every home in this huge town house complex, which I later counted was well over 60 families, had a ceiling access cover that led into the attic, which had to be a shared space to run ventilation piping, plumbing and electrical. It would be undetectable if I crawled into it and accessed each persons apartment through their access panel in each of their master bedroom en-suite. Even if there was some sort of fire wall it would be simple to cut a hole between the studs using a box cutter and a stud finder.. This meant I could access every suite in the whole building—well over fifty places. I would just need to drop into their bathroom, take all the jewelry they had in their bedroom, and be up and out in less than a minute. Though it would be tight, I knew it would be doable, so I decided to open the panel and see.

The walls didn't actually go all the way up to the actual ceiling but stopped at the apartment ceiling. I would be able to slide around the apartment complex and get access to everyone's master bathroom. I could swipe their jewelry unnoticed, even if they were home, because everyone keeps the jewelry in their bedrooms, and whats the likely hood they would be in their room at that time. But that would never happen because I could easily watch them every morning through the peephole in the door as they headed off to their job or the gym or the grocery store, and schedule my drop-in accordingly. I could take my time and rob a few per month over a longer period of time, but I think this one would be more of a do it once and hit as many places as possible all at once. I knew this would work, but was it worth it to contradict my moral compass by stealing from people who worked hard to have nice things? Was it right for me to take them from them just because I was having a hard go at life? It was with this in mind that I decided it would be better to steal something that wouldn't hurt or harm anyone specifically, either physically or financially. The thought of taking someone's jewelry was hard to justify but the thought of possibly taking someone's family heirloom that was passed down to them generation after generation was not something I could do. I know one day my family will be passed down what I feel is priceless and I couldn't imagine those ever being taken by someone that doesn't know the story behind it.

I needed to take it to the next level and had a great new idea. An idea where if planned properly I would attain everything I needed in one big score, which involved using a large magnet. I knew what I was going to do! I was going to rob a jewelry store in the mall.

It took a while to plan it but knowing what I learned about the flaw in the townhouse planning, I knew there is a flaw is almost everything, I just had to find it, so I devised what I thought was an ingenious plan! I researched the price of magnets on the internet, and we were in business. Thinking back, I believe the magnet with the 150-pound lifting capacity was $35, and a 700-pound magnet was about $79. The new plan was to wear a women's burqa that covered everything but my eyes, walk into the men's or women's bathroom in the local mall and, from there, gain access to the space between the ceiling tiles and actual roof., I would literally just be hanging out up there until after closing before making my move. I would access the ceiling about two hours before closing and just wait until later in the night. I figured because all the video cameras were on the paneled ceiling or walls and directed down, not up, I would be in the clear! With having previously saved the exact GPS locations of the jewelry display counters, all I would have to do was shimmy above that exact location and drop magnets from the celling onto the glass cabinets. That would smash the glass and all I would have to do was swing the magnet a bit, pull up the magnets, and pull off the gold and silver rings. Then all I would have to do was go up through the access panel in the actual roof where I would be home free without being seen by anyone. Then I would jump on the bus wearing the burqa (the same way I arrived to the mall) and head home.

But there was a major problem I hadn't even considered, one so big that it made me abandon the idea as soon as I found out. After buying the magnets, I tested them out on my wedding ring and found out the hard way that gold is not magnetic! But, honestly, I knew deep down it wouldn't work all along. The idea to use a vacuum went through my head for a split second, but how the hell was I to get a vacuum into the ceiling along with myself? And then what? Run down the street with a vacuum in hand? That's a funny thought, but so not realistic.

Looking back, I had many ideas had run through my head since the time I was told I was terminally ill, but the only time I really wasn't thinking of how to pull off a crime was when we went on that trip across Canada. After the trip, my thoughts went directly back to that, and I had some amazing ideas. Then I stumbled onto the perfect plan.

Though I am considered disabled, I didn't really feel that I had any restrictions when it came to planning what crime to commit. I knew that the option of riding up on a motorbike and jumping on the back of a Brinks truck with a brick of explosives was off the table. But there were many more options to pick from. I like to think that my body is just a shell casing that protects the only real living thing inside it, which is the brain. I knew the brain controls everything: touch, smell, sight, taste, and hearing. I knew this vital part of my body was fine, and that it was the only part that mattered. If the feeling sensors in your fingers are dead, there's no electrical signal going to the brain, and the brain just doesn't receive that signal of touch. But there is nothing wrong with the brain. If the feeling sensors start to work a couple of days later, it would be like you replaced a burnt-out headlight. So maybe in the future they will have a way to reconstruct my face and give me a futuristic tongue that lets me talk and taste again. But until then, I will just put an under-construction sign across my jaw area and not rely on speech or endurance to pull off a crime. I knew I needed to use stealth, or a motor, to make it happen, because running was out of the question, though I knew I could possibly use my imperfections to my advantage. Like if I was to use a really good recording of another person's voice over the phone, and there was no way I could be a suspect having no tongue and all. Just because I was different, I didn't feel disabled when it came to what I could pull off.

CHAPTER 37

The Criminal Mind

Like any normal person looking to make some quick money, I thought, *I am going to rob a bank*. I'm sure we have all thought of this at some point in our lives, even down to the detail of how exactly we were going to do it, because our mind wanders in those directions from the movies we have watched or the news we have read. We like to think, *If I were them, I would have done this differently or planned the getaway that way*. I recall watching a movie when I was a kid, in which some bank robbers kidnapped the branch manager at night in his house and the next day robbed the bank by having the branch manager let them in early in the morning right before they were to open.. Though it was a good story, it wasn't something I was capable of doing. So I started off thinking that if I was going to try to pull off this kind of job, I would start off with more of a note-style robbery, asking them to empty all the registers. I also recall the stories about Billy the Kid, who I believe also robbed some banks. Then there was Robin Hood, who stole from the rich and gave to the poor. I'm not sure he robbed banks, but he did do what he knew was wrong (though for the right reason, or so he thought). So I felt like it was justified because I was going to do something wrong but for the right reason: my family!

But reality set in as I lay in my bed and knew I should at least figure out a way to leave them with no financial burdens related to me and my death. I probably wasn't going to pull off a bank heist, large scale robbery of over 50 places in a day, or jewelry store heist, especially without knowing anyone to help me plan it. As I lay in the bed, all I could focus on was how bad a burden I was to my family. And even though I now had life insurance, dying from cancer was not going to pay out anything because I purchased it after I was diagnosed. I remembered that after we sold almost everything off, we still had a holiday camper and truck we were still paying for. If we were to sell those, we would have taken a loss, which meant we would have had to make a lump payment to the bank on the day we sold them. And we didn't have anything else to sell to be able to pay off the difference. So we were still having to make the monthly payments, which were a huge financial strain.

So I thought, *What if I drove my truck and camper straight into an oncoming train or off a bridge, making it look like an accident?* That's where these thoughts all really stemmed from. Committing suicide, but making it look like it was some sort of medical problem, like I passed out on the tracks or something. Then I thought of others and figured that would probably hurt many people if I hit a train, or what if someone drowned trying to save me from driving off a bridge? That was the last thing I wanted. I didn't want to go out in a blaze of glory that took down other people. I wanted it to be something so simple that it would involve just a quick signature on a piece of paper as just another shitty incident that took someone's life. That way, my insurance would simply pay out my family some money, which could help with the funeral costs. I was hoping the camper and truck would just be a write-off through insurance somehow. But most of all, I didn't actually want to die from cancer. I wanted to die on my own terms! It wasn't the best plan but it was an option if all was lost because it was simple and reachable

For that plan to work, I knew all I had to be able to do was get out of bed and drive. I knew I had to keep fighting to beat this … not to live for the rest of my life, but to make a plan to fix the burden I was putting on the family. So let's call that Plan B.

My plan B for my end-of-life finale was a long trip with the truck and trailer to Alberta's Badlands, where there are high drop-offs into large crevasses that any inexperienced driver (or sickly cancer victim) could easily drive down too fast and, on a sharp turn, go through a barrier and fall long enough that would turn the holiday trailer and truck into toothpicks upon impact. Insurance would pay out the trailer and truck, my life insurance would pay the accidental death, and I would die on my own terms. Sadly, in my angered state, I thought, *Why not get back at someone I fucking hated and fuck him over while doing what I had to do?*

That thought process started when I had more energy and started to think about how I would never get the chance for revenge against that guy who messed up my car and the bond I had with my dad. My thought processes and the scary ideas I had became almost sadistic. I was going to really fuck up his life like he fucked up mine. The guy (Malady) who took a shit in my car was going to get set up for murder! I have watched so many forensic TV shows and movies, and all they've shown me was that it's really hard to murder someone and get away with it, especially if you're not physically fit or trained with any kind of fighting skills. But to make a suicide look like a murder? That's a different story.

It's not what you know—it's what you can prove, and it would be easy to prove that a cancer victim had wanted to confront his high school bully, that things had gotten out of hand, and that he had killed me. It wouldn't be that hard to develop a list of clues that would support my confronting him, and in the heat of the moment, things taking a turn for the worse. All people would believe is that the guy who already had previous charges as an accomplice to murder

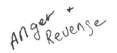

would kill again in a fit of rage. I would have to use my social media accounts to say I was going to confront him, break a window to get into his house, and continue to break a couple more things to set the scene for that heart-stopping surprise when the police broke down the door after I called 911 and asked for help as he trapped me in his apartment. I'd yell, in my muffled voice, "He's trying to kill me! He's got a knife." I would have time to end my life on my own terms, he would be screwed for life, and my family would get the insurance money, as I wouldn't have died from cancer. I would/could have done it in such a way that I would not feel the pain of my skin getting sliced open, because there are many spots on my body (more specifically my neck) that due to the surgeries, I have no feeling. So it could be done painlessly too. The only thing I would need to do was ensure I did this during a time that he would have no alibies. Like when he walks his dog or buy figuring out a way to get him out of the house like setting up a fake meeting with an old high school buddy or whatever

He wouldn't actually be there leaving his fingerprints on the murder weapons at the time, but most likely they will have already been there before because its his house. I would use two knives from the kitchen Everything would point to him doing it, and, with a few well-placed towels and cleaner spilled on the floor, it would look like he had been in the middle of hiding the evidence when he heard the cops and made a run for it. When they caught him without his ever knowing what even happened, his life would be fucked. Or at least fucked over for a few years while he was in jail and trying to fight through court. He would just deny that he knew what they were talking about, which is what every guilty man says. I could throw his life into a complete disaster in a flip of a switch, And the best thing about it was I could do this at any time, making the decision of when I was ready to die even more my own.

206

There isn't much preparation required to execute this plan besides some expression of my inner rage on my social media account that I had to get off my chest before facing this end-of-life decision. All I would have to do was wait to see him leave his place and break in right after. I would do it then because, that way, when they started searching for him after the cops got there, he would literally be fleeing the crime scene without his even knowing it. Any alibi he had wouldn't be of any use, because the arrival time of wherever Malady was headed would be too close to call. As for the exact time I died, it would have been estimated, not exact to the minute making it even a harder case for him to prove himself innocent.

It would be like killing two birds with one stone: my family gets the insurance money, and I get my revenge. I had a sadistic new plan, but regardless of the dangerous mind this dying man had, my short-term goals needed to be reached before anything could come to fruition. I needed to get my sorry, self-pitied ass out of bed and start lining things up.

After I started getting more energy, I kept wavering back and forth between plans as I figured I must be able to do a little better than just getting enough money to pay off some vehicles. The amount I would get from insurance really wasn't enough for my family to survive long term, I needed to get enough money to cover more than just paying off a few debts, and I really liked the idea of the magnet robbery. But I still didn't have the mobility to get into the ceiling, let alone the fact that jewelry wasn't magnetic. So how about I rob a bank? I returned to this early idea, thinking, *What if I was to actually rob a bank?* Would I slip a note to the teller, with guns a-blazing? Like I said earlier, there was no real punishment for me, regardless of what law I broke, as my outcome was already foretold. So this was my last chance to ensure the financial survival of my family. I was thinking that at the busiest time in the bank, I would write a note telling the teller that I had five other accomplices in the bank that were casually walking around, waiting for my signal, and that they were also armed. It would also say that we would lock down the bank and kill one random person every 240 seconds. I would demand $300,000 in cash and say that once we had it, we'd be gone. I would flash a gun, or something that looked like a gun, and as she was processing everything in her head, right in front of her face I would start my stopwatch counting down from 240 seconds. If she didn't call my bluff and we got to the point where the money was on the counter, I would hand across the last note that said we would walk out quietly one at a time to ensure she didn't call the cops or trip the silent alarm. That way, she wouldn't know who was still watching her. At the bottom of each note I would ask her to nod if she understood. As talking was not something I wanted her to hear, so she couldn't pinpoint me in any other way besides my average height. That went through my head until reality set in. What if she called my bluff? And not only would I never hurt innocent people, I would probably hate myself for causing an unnecessary trauma to someone who didn't deserve it. There are already so many bad things in this world that people see all the time—why scare them more by making them suffer life-altering experiences, regardless of whether it's fake or not? So I totally went a different route and dropped the whole bank robbery idea.

Then I started to think about an idea that was more of a grab and go. But the problem with thefts like robberies and breaking and entering is that it's hard to hide evidence. So why not rob them on a larger scale. Instead of trying to figure out a way to sneak into a building and break/crack the code on a safe just make a plan, where you take the whole damn safe and destroy everything at once. Basically, completely destroy the building, steal the safe, and figure out a way to open it when you're in the clear. By this point it was very noticeable that my energy level was improving.

I thought, *What skills do I have? What tools do I have access to? Who do I know who would help me, knowing how desperate I am and my situation?* I thought, *I do own a large one-ton diesel truck that can pull almost anything down the highway.* This particular crime would have to be executed in the summer so I wouldn't need to deal with unpredictable weather like icy roads or snow drifts. I wondered what I could steal that is easily accessible, can be found in a lot of random places, and could cause a lot of damage and help me steal a safe. It occurred to me that we often see road crews with heavy equipment and excavators on the side of the road who don't work weekends. I knew my truck could pull big machinery, so I came up with a plan to use that to my advantage.

. Most robbers don't want to be seen. They want to get in and out as quickly and quietly as possible, hoping no one ever realizes someone was there. Well, this was the exact opposite of that! Knowing my best friend and how loyal we are to each other, I knew if I asked him to help me commit a crime, he would do it without question—or at the very least, he would supply me with whatever I needed, and in this case, I would need an accomplice. If I said I was helping him at the farm, and he confirmed it, I would be in the clear. Our loyalty to each other is beyond the law. We are brothers who sleep in separate houses, brothers who had different sisters, and we are each other's family. But if he refused for whatever reason, I knew him so well I could easily convince him to help me, because if he didn't, he would have to witness my family being ripped apart financially and watch his niece and nephew suffer. Luckily for me, the path that he followed in life was to become one of the best heavy equipment operators I have ever known, which would be essential for this plan to work. He had given years of dedication to his job and worked under all kinds of conditions. He could make those excavators move around like a ballet dancer. Without exaggeration, it's pure grace watching him move those masses of metal around with such precision and delicacy. But even more importantly what I remembered the most about his job, from years back, was him telling me that all the keys for each name brand of excavator were the same key cut , meaning if you had a key to a CAT excavator, you had a key to *all* CAT excavators—John Deere, Kamatsu, etc. So here is what I came up with: a plan I called Digger D.

We would use my truck and drive to a staging place for government-run construction crews that worked Monday to Friday. I would hook onto a trailer that had a piece of machinery on it ready for transport—and in Alberta, they are all around. We would wear all the proper PPE and have a beacon light on so as not to cause suspicion, as it would look like a normal highway road crew thing. I would do this on a Friday night, about 11:00 p.m. and have him call in a drunk driver or something to distract the police while we set up. If the machinery was already loaded and the tracks were chained, it could be hitched up in fewer than four minutes. We would drive it out of town to our hiding spot, where we would gear up and get ready for the night. We would ensure the bucket was free to move around and keep the tracks chained and then put on our gear. Here, we would also change the plates of the truck if we hadn't done so already. We would have our route planned out to each business or a place where we knew we could get a big score at a company that had a huge safe, jewelry case or an ATM machine, or something along those lines. Next, I would drive to the side of the building where there would be no video cameras, because we would only hit places with cameras facing the front or back doors and/or windows. With my friend already in the excavator as it was running, I would stop the truck and hop into the bucket of the machine, geared up with chains and a radio. He would push the bucket right through the wall and open it up. While wearing all black and a full-face mask, I would pop out like the Easter Bunny on steroids and direct him to grab onto the safe with the claw of the machine, or swing side to side to break the jewelry display cases or whatever necessary for the specific target we chose to hit. If a safe was not within reach of the bucket, I would wrap a chain around it and use the machine to pull it out. Once it was out, he would scoop the safe into the bucket, wrap the arm back in to move it, and we would be on the road within one or three minutes. We would do this in a town that didn't have its own police station, giving us more time to get away. Next, we would get back to the hiding place, where we would use the power of the machine to claw open the lock of the safe, then head back to the construction site where we'd put the trailer and machinery back in place and drive home. So even if they knew they were looking for a massive machine, the people that had the actual excavator that was used in the crime, would have no reason to even report it as missing, making it even harder for the cops to solve. If they ever even figured out the machine that had been used, it would be a government one, and who knew how many city workers had access to that machine? I was really into this and was working out the details every day as my battle continued when I came to the realization that I should aim for something more realistic. When I was thinking about it and making the plans, I realized that this plan was all based around *my friend's* skillset. But how could I put that kind of pressure on him, even if he was the best for the job? If the machine gets caught in the rubble, for even a few minutes that could mean the end of my freedom with no pay out.

The truth of it was, it was the perfect crime for *him* to commit, but what did *I* know and what could *I* do that would capitalize on my skillset? A desperate man is willing to rob someone but most likely will get caught, but why? Because he doesn't know the systems, protocols, or security measures he's dealing with. So instead of doing something crazy, like demolishing a building to steal a safe, why didn't I use what I knew, which was working in a corporate office? I knew exactly what form goes where, what division processes what, and what computer systems talk to each other. I could easily find some flaws in the system—like how the excavators are all keyed the same, or that certain IDs don't have pictures, or something along those lines—and use them to my advantage. So I focused on finding flaws in as many systems as possible and trying to figure out a way to link them to make an untraceable robbery.

It's not every day you look back on your life and recognize your mistakes and regrets and have to dwell and hang on to them. But I had nothing else to distract me from my thoughts, so I did that constantly. At this point, I reached a new low in my life. I was desperate and full of hatred toward anyone and everyone. I had only my small circle of people I wanted to protect and was willing to do anything for them. That's when things all changed for me. I had my second encounter with my spiritual guide, my God. It's impossible to explain if you haven't experienced this, but your body fills with a temperature-less warmth and a peacefulness that can't be put into words. I like to think that from that point forward, things had taken a turn for the better, and I had to come up with a way to give back to people.

I started writing my story down for my kids to learn more about their dad and who I was growing up, but in the end realized I should share it for all to learn from my lessons and experiences so they could know what was to come if they were in the same situation, and/or for unknowing people to know what a person's mind may go through on their deathbed. They only want to be remembered and not forgotten. That's really why people get gravestones, to forever have an acknowledgement that they existed. Because, really, every moment is a memory, and every memory is a moment. This expression planted a seed of an idea that flourished over the years. God wants my story to be heard, because I can revolutionize how we remember our loved ones and ensure their voice is heard long after they are gone. I was to live so I could give people the opportunity to move onto the next stage knowing they will not be forgotten, thus helping the transition to be more peaceful and less scary for them and their loved ones.

Now what He asked of me comes at no little cost to me. I thought everything I had overcome was the hardest thing I would face, but the hardest was yet to come—to open my heart and mind fully to my savior and trust that things were all meant to happen this way, and all for a specific reason. Getting rid of the anger and hatred and repairing the morally ripped fibers out of me would take time. My hardest hurdle was finding the trust in Him to follow His advice and know it would work out in the end. Everything that has happened has made me more than cautious about who I let into my life, and who to believe is there to help me. So it was very hard for me to believing in something I saw some weird day that I knew wasn't physically there, telling me it would be OK and to follow the direction He suggested because it would work out for me if I did, as He said it would. When I looked at it from a more rational perspective, it sounded like the immunotherapy was giving me hallucinations or the start of a secondary personality disorder.

I needed more persuading to believe that this inner voice was my God. And I couldn't believe what happened next. I would have liked to be able to say I opened my heart to God that day, but the truth is, I wasn't so sure. He didn't give up trying to get through to me. There were many more of these moments when my brain would connect on a totally different level and I would have these intense conversations with whom I can only say was myself, in my mind, kind of like we connected in a form of telepathy. Even on what was to be the sunniest of days, it takes time for the fog to lift before the sun can shine through. It would take many of these "conversations" before we created a bond of trust with one another. But funny, insignificant things started to happen, and over time, I realized that everything was aligning, and I started to see how the dots were connecting and the direction this was all aimed toward. These moments would present themselves and things would just happen and work out, and every piece of the puzzle would come together. As I write this, I am in a great state of mind knowing I can throw the sheets to the wind and see where this ride takes us. I am along for the ride in this strategic plan that has been set for me.

Health-wise, I was getting so much better, and the cancer was shrinking by the day from the immunotherapy. It was a hell of an uphill battle, but it was working. My wife graduated from dental hygiene school and, all of a sudden, the chains broke free and we could live anywhere in Canada we wanted (Keeping in mind I would need to travel to get to my monthly immunotherapy for life) . Because of my cancer treatments and the cost of flights, we decided to move to Nanaimo, BC. We would be close to my parents and sister and live in a natural and peaceful environment. Another big reason was its affordability versus mainland rental costs, let alone the business of the city and rush-hour traffic. So that's where we put our focus on the next stage of our lives.

For me, Toronto was a cold and dismal place, but that also has a lot to do with my attitude when I was there. I missed the friends and support system we had in Red Deer and the conversations we had with my friends on the block , from issues of raising kids and the crazy things they do, to just waving hello as you walked by. Back there, my heart was filled with love. Being able to talk about the crazy mom down the road that can't control her son to advising when to plant vegetables. That's what I was looking for, the same exact people, but on the island, where I could live in nature and near the ocean. So when my wife completed her dental hygiene course, that's where we went. Things seemed to magically work out for us as we stumbled upon a house where a mother of three had recently lost her husband and was taking off for a three-month vacation while she grieved. The house was fully furnished, which was great for us. The plan was to stay in the house for three months and not even unpack anything but our clothes. Then, in three months, Bambi would have a new job, I would be comfortable with taking the ferry once a month to my appointments, and we would buy a house using the proceeds from the sale of the Red Deer house when the rent-to-own contract was up, which was right around the corner.

We moved in and it was great—no real unpacking, just our clothes, and suddenly we were island goers! But it turned out the island wasn't all it was cracked up to be, with ferry cancelations and the very different types of people that lived there, which I don't mean in a bad way. I wasn't used to the way people were raising their kids, and the freedom they gave their children made me uncomfortable. I didn't feel it was OK to let my kids stand next to a cliff above a raging current of crashing ocean waves. I am a bit more old-fashioned when it comes to the do's and don'ts of what my kids can do. More than that, it just didn't feel right, I didn't feel home. I did have many beautiful memories of this amazing place. The outdoor setting was what you dream about—the lush trees and harmonic sunsets. I had many more "conversations" during my stay there, and we went over many things and answered many of life's questions, like what my goals were and the meaning of life and what real love is. He taught me to forgive my high school bully, whom I do forgive, for if he hadn't done what he did, I wouldn't have been fired up with the rage and strength I needed to get through this. Without him, I may not have had that extra determination to live. My new focus was to build this unorthodox relationship of trust and learn how to accept love back into my life. With so much hate, I had forgotten how to really love, and I wanted and needed to remember. Not that Bambi and I were not in love, but I was searching for the meaning of love so I could show people what it felt like to feel love, actually *feel* it. Love that is never having to second-guess a decision because it's clouded by fog, like when you walk past a bouquet of flowers and think, *My wife would love that*, but then debate if the price is too high. I don't want those clouds to follow me anymore. I want to buy the flowers regardless of the price, just to see that smile on her face and that look of surprise when you show her an act of love. I wanted her to have so much love around her that she doesn't even acknowledge it, I want the love to be so much that its just part of her every day life. I wanted to know how to rid myself of hatred and anger.

He said to let go of the wheel and let Him navigate the waters, and that's what I did. And here is what happened. While we were in Nanaimo, Bambi struggled to find a job. I mean, the job opportunities weren't as we had hoped. So we spent the entirety of our time there taking walks on the beach, talking to new people, and biking. Because school hadn't started, we finally got a bit of a break together as a family. After the three months, we decided to move to Kelowna, because there was more opportunity for Bambi to work, as she had already lined up a job prior to moving. She told me they were the nicest people and had the best office and working environment and that she was going to be great friends with them.

So that was great, as she was to start her new job and we could settle down in another shorter-term rental until we found what was to be our second forever home. The rental was nice, with an amazing view over a vineyard and a few houses up on the mountain nestled in vibrant, green fields for miles to see. I spent more time planning and organizing things, as I had nothing but time, while Bambi was at work and my kids went to school. I created an idea for a business that assists people who are dying with making their passing less scary. All I needed was laser-driven focus and a heck of a lot of trust in what I felt and know is right, because it came directly from my heart. Though I was very busy with my work, projects, and writing this book, I was desperately lonely. It was hard being in a foreign city that was a four-hour drive from family or friends. My kids were not liking their classmates because they were new to the school and were considered the odd ones out. But I was able to focus all my attention into my projects, and, funny thing, the day I finished was the same day we get a call from the rent-to-own people saying something had come up and they were moving out of our Red Deer house, and it was ours again. WHAT???? Full circle!

Life for us today is right back to how it was when we first started this whole adventure. It's like I never left and all that stuff in the past is a distant memory. Though I have the battle scars to prove it, I am sitting here as if it were all a dream. I am back in my house, sitting in my office and typing this story to you as if we never left and it was all made up. But all the pieces landed in place, as promised. I was going to hang up a picture of the family where it had hung before this whole thing started, and even the nail hole was still there as if it was just there waiting for it. We have all our friends and family close by, and our amazing friendly neighbors back on the same street we plan to grow old on. And my kids are loving their schools and friends again. Their smiles and laughter are back after having been missing for so long. Sadly, my wife misses her fellow employees from her last job, with her new career and the state of the world today (COVID-19). As one of the highest at-risk front-line workers with the potential to be exposed to the virus, she will need to be more focused on the job than ever. We are not out of the woods yet, but with the professionalism and seriousness of these key influencers in our system, we can ensure the survival of our species. They are the soldiers on our front line for preventing infection. If we all work together and do what we know is right, we should be OK by October 2021. Now that things are back to what I like to think is normal, with a few lessons learned along the way, I am able to pass on my experiences and knowledge of how to show your loved ones the meaning of true love. And I can begin the next stage of my life, which is to provide a service to keep a person's memory and love alive long after they have moved on to the next chapter. I created

Heavenly Messenger because I was able to listen to and follow my heart. And with the current state of the world and people dying all over without being able to have their loved ones there with them during these hard times, and not being able to spread their words of wisdom to their loved ones because they are quarantined, this service is more needed than ever before.

Heavenly Messenger was created to securely store and hold the personal messages of our loved ones *for* our loved ones. Just because people's voices may be silenced doesn't mean they can't be heard. The service provides the opportunity to share life lessons and stories and express emotions to loved ones at a future date. We want to give people the comfort and peace of mind to know that no matter what illness, tragic event, or lost time, their voice is still being heard by the ones they love the most, and they are being remembered.

And the same goes for the receiver—we want you to know that just because someone may not be physically with you, you are never truly alone, and they are there in spirit, divulging their stories and kind words for you at those special moments in life, like birthdays, anniversaries, and graduations. For so many of us, the hardest thing is coming to terms with being forgotten, so I created a system to help take that fear away. If you want to know more about it, refer to the website at the end of the book. You can track my progress through the success of the business. As my brother said, look for the good in your life's journey by bringing to light the bad—through that, you will find your calling.

Now, as promised, I need to share with you what it means to love. I am not talking about lust here, as that's a whole other thing, but true love and how to show it to the ones you care about, as well as the one you share a bed with. Love is having complete trust in and feeling protected by the one you are with, be it your dad, who will put his life on the line to ensure you feel cared for, or your mom, who helped you learn to walk and talk and was there when you were hurt or needed affection. Love can be shown in so many ways. As an example, you are heading home from work and have to stop for gas, and while you're at the gas station, you buy her one of her favorite chocolate bars. Or you mow your neighbor's lawn because you know it will save him some hard work and make him smile. Love is hosting a family barbecue for your friends and family during a pandemic while ensuring everyone keeps a good social distance so no one is exposed to unnecessary disease. Love is offering to play your sister's favorite board game on game-night when you really wanted to play yours. Love is helping your dad with the chores because you know he's feeling weak. And love is actively listening to someone about their day or problems and giving them your undivided attention and offering advice if they ask for it. Love is all around us, but if we get blinded by the fog, it can be hard to see. I was surrounded by all this love throughout my health struggles but chose not to realize it was all around me. It wasn't until I opened my heart to the unknown, and I am so much happier for this and so is my family. Yours will be too if you open your heart to the world and love around you.

The last lesson I want to share is a hard one to talk about when it comes to love. This is the love between two people in an intimate relationship. I lost this for years, as I was totally insecure about my looks and my body, having a trachea, stomach tube, distorted lower jaw, and bulbus chin. But I was stupid to think my looks actually mattered. It's not about me and my insecurities; it's about her, as the love between you and this person is not just physical but emotional. This is the person you rush to talk to about the amazing news you have when you are told you beat cancer, and the person you talk to when something awful and unexpected happens in your life. This is the person you can openly cry in front of and share your emotions and feelings with, without guilt.

Zack, you need to know this next part for when you're older and married, and same goes for you, Kisenya. Zack you need to know this to know how to really treat your wife and Kisenya, this is how you need to be treated and how you show love to your partner in a physical way. For this, you will need time to prep and plan. Lust is spontaneous, but truly showing love is properly thought out. Like you have learned from me, the quality of the wrapping is just as important as the present itself, and the same goes for love. The first thing you need to do is set the time and place and, of course, prepare. This includes showing her your thoughtfulness and reminding her of her beauty. The day before, schedule her into a spa for a beauty nail thing or some sort of pampering that makes them feel special and pretty. It's not like I care about that stuff, but I want her to feel her sexiest and flawless in the moment. With this done the day before, she won't feel like she's been caught off guard, with her body not being prepared. The last thing you want is for them to feel like they are not up to your expectation in the moment. It's about her feeling comfortable with you in the moment. The best time would be just after a long day at work, when I know she is at her most stressed, and you drop a bomb of relaxation and tranquility to a long day at work. Show he you have everything handled and the rest of the day is all about her. My idea of the perfect setting would be to scatter rose petals up the stairs and into the bathroom so that she walks into a setting of tranquility. Only you will know what your partner would appreciate if you truly know them. Some may think a garage-type setting involving their truck is sexy, while others may like a backyard, outdoorsy setting. Each person is different, and only if you truly know and love them can you know what they want. But the basis for all this is the same, and here you will learn your final and most important lesson from me.

Like I said, the setting needs to be what makes them happy and comfortable. For me, perfect presentation and suspenseful build-up would be the walk she would take from the door along a trail of rose petals into the master bedroom bathroom. There would be a hint of the smell of my cologne combined with the smell of the outside fresh air as it would slightly breeze through the house. As she passes through the bedroom, she would see it romantically decorated, like you would in a luxury hotel room. As she makes her way through the bedroom while still following the rose path, she would look into the large bathroom and see the perfect décor lit by flickering candle light, making it seem like she was in a spa or extravagant resort. She would see a steaming bubble bath under a candlelit ambiance. The combination of a few new ferns, the fragrance of her favorite bubble bath, and the flicker of the candlelight will set the mood for what's to come. She will undress herself in the comfort of her own silky skin and then slide into the steaming pool of tranquility and let all the stresses of the day melt into the humidity of the room. There would be a small present on the side of the bathtub, and the card would say, "We have all night, so take you time and enjoy the moment." The gift would say on it, "Do not open until you're done in the bath." After a few minutes of relaxation, silence, and peace, I would play a song from the record player in our room, one to help her to melt into the moment ("Your Song" by Elton John). I would have a list of romantic, calming songs that would play for as long as she wanted to hear them. Once done, she would open the gift, which would not be anything slutty or uncomfortable, but a nice silky, sexy, comfortable piece of thin-fabric clothing that accentuates the curves of her beautiful body. This must be sexy and classy to make her feel enchanting. Make sure when she walked out that you acknowledged all the beauty she has to offer; you need to show her that you think of her as the most precious, amazing, smart, sexy, beautiful woman you have ever seen. In this moment it is only the two of you, no outside distractions., like you are the last two people on earth. Make her comfortable and take things very, very slowly. You have all night with her, so if you want her to feel your love, you need to ensure it lasts so she has many memories and experiences in this strategically choreographed event. Let her get comfortable and stop the music. This will show her that this is a not a spontaneous moment but a planned event that showcases her as the centerpiece of your masterpiece. Then, once she is comfortable, I would start the playlist to set the stage for act two. This music, with candles flickering in the darkness of the bedroom and the smell of roses and her silky skin from the bath, will have enticed three of her senses. The slight flutter of the candles will trigger her sight to an almost illusionary form, and the smell will trigger her sense of beauty and cleanliness in its fragrance, while the music enlightens the moment to almost glorify the whole performance. From here, I entice the sense of taste with some chocolate-covered strawberries to trigger one of the last senses before moving on to the sense of touch.

You don't do what most men do by skipping to the final act of the performance. From here, you need to savor every moment, touch, and sound. Take it all in with her and become as romantic as you've ever wished to be. Slow things down with a shoulder massage or foot rub and explore every sensory receptor on her body. Use the songs' length to know where you are in your act, and after exploring the love of your life's body and triggering every one of her senses to a point of almost explosion-ary eroticism, you can move into act three. I won't elaborate here, but basically if you did everything right, you can let your animalistic urges take over and become one with each other. That is how you show proper physical love with your partner. But the key factor that needs to take place, regardless of how perfect or flawed your performance was, is showing her your continued interest in her afterward with intimate conversation or cuddling. Don't just roll over and fall asleep. Like any masterpiece, this one needs its artist to come back on stage for his applause. And if you really want to surprise the audience, you finish with an encore!

CHAPTER 38

To Conclude

Please note, I am far from perfect, as you have found out. I have had my ups and downs in life, and there are many things I would change if I could, like being a better son to my parents, a better husband to my wife, and not getting so caught up in things like work and money where I miss out on special moments, like watching the kids play together and laugh. Those are the moments I took for granted. But I don't want to anymore.

What I regret most that I never saw at the time was that I wasn't around for my family when they needed me the most, like when my mom went through breast cancer, or when my kids asked "Where's Daddy?" When I was away for months at a time. They of course did not understand why I had to leave, or the concept of money yet. All they knew was that Daddy saw them for a couple of days and then left for a long, long time. I would have hated to learn they were wondering the whole time what they'd done wrong to make Daddy so mad that he didn't want to see them anymore. For that reason, I am grateful I got cancer, because if I hadn't, I wouldn't have been able to be the man I am today. I wouldn't have had all this time with my family, making an unbreakable bond of respect and trust. I won't ever leave my kids again just to make money if it means I won't be able to be there for them at a moment's notice if they need me. My kids are an extension of me, partly my body, mind, and soul. They are the best of me and their mom combined. I was an idiot who didn't see what I was doing to them and how terrible that must have been on them and Bambi for all those years when I was at work and when I was so mad at the world. I truly feel the real reason that God gave me a second chance was that He wanted me to see the true value in life, as I completely missed it the first time around. This time, I won't fuck it up. I will be at their side through everything, thick and thin, for the rest of my dying days. My kids can count on Mommy and Daddy as a united team to help them through any uphill battles they may face.

Bambi, there is something special I did just for you because I love you so much and appreciate everything you've done for me, and for what you are doing for our family. I want to make your every wish come true, so before I give you that gift, I wanted to throw the sheets to the wind and give my Hail Mary shout-out to Ellen DeGeneres to please ask Bambi Kom-Tong to come meet you on your show and fulfill one of the boxes on her life long bucket list. Ellen, with your permission, I would love for my wife to meet you and full fill a dream of hers that I was not able to yet full fill, by having her see you on your show. Maybe she would be able to come to your show and present to all your viewers and the world her story and what I have created to help ease people into an easier transition. I'm sure Bambi will be a fun guest for you, as she loves playing games but loses like a spoiled sport, and I'm sure she can elaborate on any of these stories, like how she conned me into having to swim with a big fish to make my baby smarter. Bambi deserves a moment in the spotlight for what she has done, put up with, and put on the line throughout the years. If you are reading this, Ellen, help me out on this one please. I will owe you a solid!

Bambi, if you are reading this for the first time, my final wish is to make sure all your wishes come true. You have spent more than your fair share of time looking after me when any other person in their right mind would have given up. Your drive and persistence have kept me alive, whether it was pushing me to take the extra step or nursing me when I wasn't capable of doing it on my own. You ensured I never gave up, even though I wanted to many times. You have done way more than anything you were obligated to as a wife. There are no words that can express how grateful I am to have you as my partner. And though I can't promise that things will ever be normal again, I will do everything in my power to ensure you know how much I appreciate you and what you did for this family. You not only sacrificed your time and dreams, but you did this all while ensuring I never saw you weak, as you knew if I saw you fall apart, I would be right behind you falling apart too. I can't believe the strength you had to do this all on your own. No one will ever really know the shit you had to go through and the weight of the world you had on your shoulders. So, for this, I will spend every last breath doing what I can to make your dreams come true. And knowing that one of the items on your bucket list is to meet Ellen, I worked that into my plans to be a squeaky wheel and pray for it to happen. If you are not my wife reading this, please take a moment to send Ellen a message to see if you can get her on the show! Bambi, as for the other items on your bucket list—like going to Egypt and riding a camel—I will do everything in my power to stay alive until I can make that happen for you. But one thing at a time.

CHAPTER 39

To My Kids And Wife

Kids, please continue with your taekwondo. This skill will teach you confidence and discipline, and you should never have to live in fear like I did. As you have already read, this ruined so many things and caused so many years of anger and regret. Fear and lack of confidence held me back from my true potential, so there is no way in hell I will let that happen to you two! Zack and Kisenya, I know how amazing you are and that you will change the world. You will both become whatever you want. You have the brains to do anything in this world, and I know you will accomplish all your life's goals! When you grow up, you will make a real difference. With your mother's amazing outlook on survival/never giving up, her determination and drive, and how she always sees the good in people, I know you two will make a positive change in this world! You know how I know this? I know for a fact that my kids are smarter than most kids out there ... because of the dolphins. LOL LOL LOL LOL. (Damn it, Bambi, those damn dolphins!) Kids, Daddy will always be here to support you, and I will never steer you wrong. I will fight any battles you face right by your side. You know that I love you both with all my heart and will use every last breath to provide you with everything you need to have a successful and fulfilling life. If anything goes wrong, I need you to know I love you so much, but I want and need you guys not to be saddened by this. With what I have created, I will be there with you, helping to create a memory for us to share in every major step of your lives. My presence will be known and my voice will still be heard at your weddings, graduations, and even during your first break-ups. Knowing we are truly happy back in our home with our family and friends here to support us is exactly how I hoped things would be again. Knowing you are safe at home with your mom, who can now take on the burden of all financial responsibilities, and that you will have the lives and opportunities intended for you, completely warms my heart. I now know you will all be OK without me if I am to move on, and my memory will now live on and I can die a happy man. They say the cancer is now gone and that my life can return back to normal, but with everything I have been through my life will never be back to normal. I see things in a new light and every new bump, mole or cut brings that fear back that I will have to face it all again. Just this time with Heavenly Messenger, I will be way more prepared.

To the Reader

Family and our kids are the most important people in our lives, and when we are all six feet under (or turned into a diamond, like I want), pictures and memories will be all that's left. I want my kids to remember the fun they had with me and the things I was able to show and teach them. I want the best for all the ones I love, and I want you all to get the very best in life. Don't let fear hold you back from doing something that's right or that you love—and if you want people to listen, make sure your voice is heard. I want you guys to reach for the stars and get closer than anyone ever has in this world. Remember, every moment will become a memory, so how do you want to be remembered and more importantly how do you want to remember yourself? As someone that did everything they could to enjoy their life, or as someone lost in a fog? That choice is yours to make. I just hope my stories were able to shed some light on some of my mistakes so that you could learn from them and not take for granted the things and people we have in our lives. I hope I helped to shed some light on the love we have surrounding us. We live by our moral compass and will not change or budge for anyone. We are Kom-Tongs and we are leaders. With sincere love in my heart, I want to tell you I love you. And I want to thank you all for spending the time reading my story and understanding why I did what I did. I hope you will forgive me if this affected you negatively in any way!

Though this is the end of this book, this is far from the end of the story. I am in the final stages of launching the Heavenly Messenger Inc. business. After my encounter with death, I knew I had to dedicate myself to helping people cope with the inevitability of being forgotten as if they were never there. I came up with a solution to ensure your voice is heard long after you have been silenced. With what I created, you can still send a message to your kid on their birthday and give them life altering advice during their life-altering moments. Though you may experience the moments in different time zones, so to speak, you will still share them. Like I said, there is much more to the story, as we are just getting started! Come check us out at www.heavenly-messenger.com

Lastly and most importantly, to my gorgeous wife, who has the strength and will of a warrior. Bambi, I can't find a more fitting way to end my book than this. You inspire me every day and make me strive to be a better and stronger person. Though there are a lot of people I look up to and who inspire me, you are always the one I look up to the most. I need you to know that my story and life are indebted to you for always being by my side, battling everything life has thrown at us, fighting for me when I couldn't fight for myself.

Long before we ever met, you poured your heart out in a wonderfully expressive poem that touches my heart every time I read it. My gift to you and the end to this story is showing and publishing your work, as it needs to be on display for the world to read.

CHAPTER 40

Bambi's Poem (Life)

LIFE:

By Bambi-Jane Sheppard (2004), aka Bambi-Jane Kom-Tong

Life is a nightmare
You can say that it is never fair
You work as hard as you do
And still no-one pays attention to you
You work hard and earn people's respect
And still they get your name incorrect
You feel alone in this place
What you really need is a loving embrace
But no one has the time anymore
You are standing right outside their door
Dripping wet from the cold rain
Their abuse is driving you insane
It's not physical but verbal instead
And now you are hanging on by a thin thread
There's only one person who can help you now
But I can only help you if you allow
The whole of your existence is based on a single string.
When it breaks who will reel you in?

PICTURES

Life As I Know It

Shielded From Realities Of Life

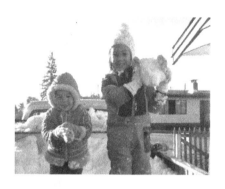

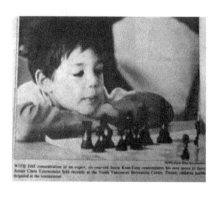

WITH THE concentration of an expert, six-year-old Jason Kim-Fung contemplates his next move at the Junior Chess Tournament held recently at the North Vancouver Recreation Centre. Twenty children participated in the tournament.

20 - Wednesday, March 23, 1994 - North Shore News

SPORTS

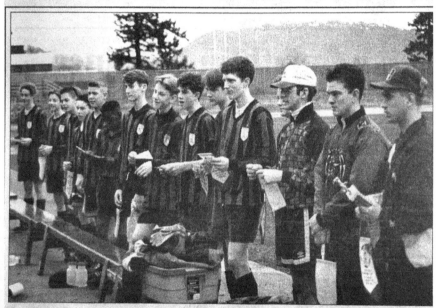

Photo submitted

MEMBERS OF the Lions Gate Falkirks were all smiles as they received awards for a 2-0 victory over the Killarney Thunder in Burrard Cup action earlier this month at Swangard Stadium in Burnaby. The under-16 team from North Vancouver, coached by Lorna Hareruk and Jeff Bolton, was one of five North Shore squads that competed in the annual soccer tournament.

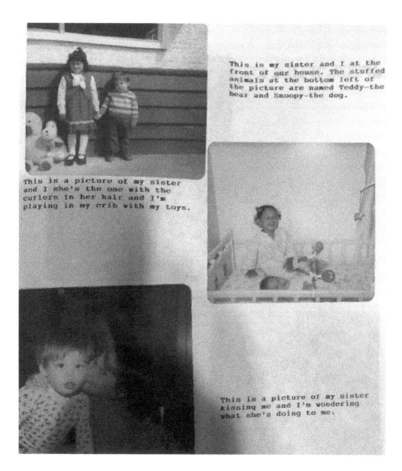

This is my sister and I at the front of our house. The stuffed animals at the bottom left of the picture are named Teddy-the bear and Snoopy-the dog.

This is a picture of my sister and I she's the one with the curlers in her hair and I'm playing in my crib with my toys.

This is a picture of my sister kissing me and I'm wondering what she's doing to me.

Following Your Path

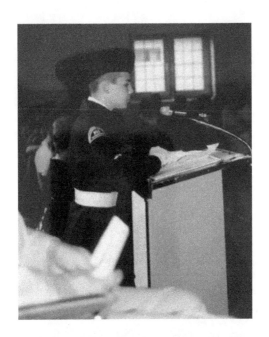

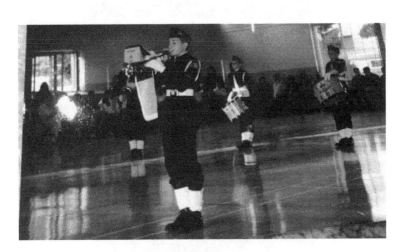

When Dreams Die, New Beginnings Start

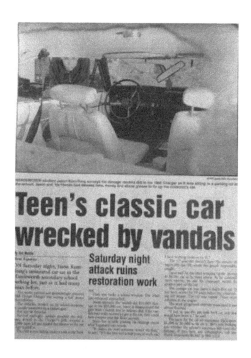

Teen's classic car wrecked by vandals

Saturday night attack ruins restoration work

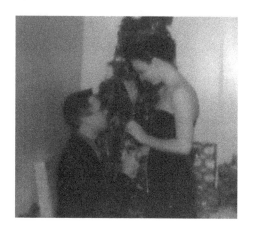

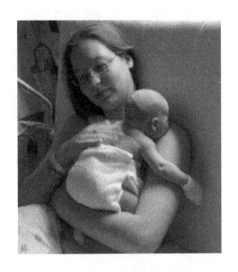

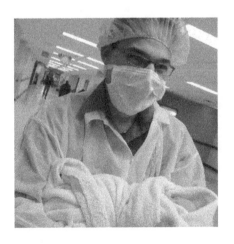

Places Your Mind Can Take You

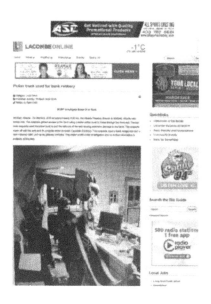

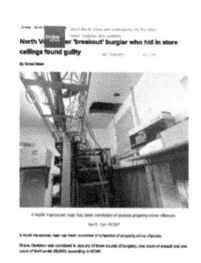

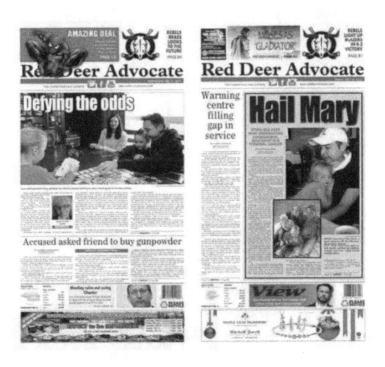

Preparing For Life

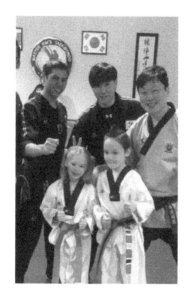
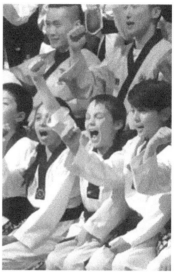

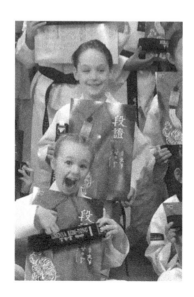

Knowing Your Calling

Mission Statement:

Though you may be silenced, We at Heavenly Messenger will ensure your voice is still heard.

Companies Goal:

To enable our customers the opportunity to divulge life lessons, stories and emotions to their loved ones at a future date & time. We want to give people the comfort and piece of mind of them knowing no matter an illness, tragic event or lost time, their voice is still being heard by the ones they love the most.

Mission:

At Heavenly Messenger our mission is to provide a professional, secure, reliable service for all our customers in a very user-friendly manner. Our service enables our customers to create messages for their loved ones, which we then store at a secure facility on their behalf for the allotted period of time. On the requested release date, we will then ensure their message gets sent out for delivery to the customers chosen recipient.

President

Jason Kom-Tong

www.heavenly-messenger.com

Unbreakable Bonds

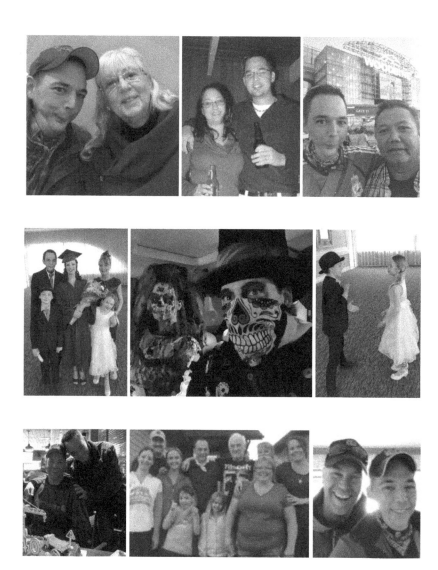

Adapting To Our New Reality

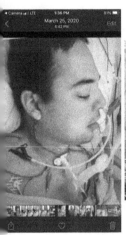
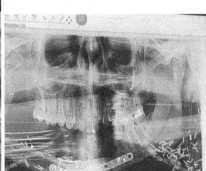
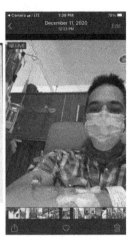

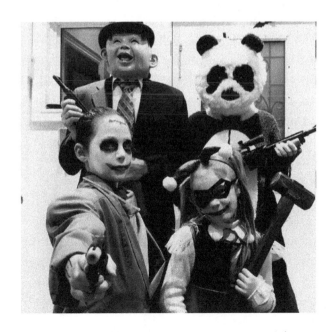

END OF NOTES

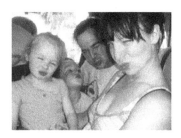

The Dangerous Mind of a Dying Man is about my memories, thoughts, lessons, and decisions, spanning from when I was a typical kid growing up to becoming a successful businessman, to the whole shit show that happened before, during, and after lying on my deathbed. My story/life is being told to you exactly how I remember, with the exception of a few peoples names for obvious reasons. This is not a history book of the exact way things happened because there are always two sides to every story, so I can only tell my side of the story and my views. Looking back at my life and how I chose to experience it, I learned how I needed to live my second shot at life and rise to the top again.

The Dangerous Mind of a Dying Man shows how the mind can force you to travel to many different places without ever having to move an inch, and how your life can be flipped upside down with no contributing known factor. What road will you decide to follow if you are told you had only three months to live? What would you change in your life? Who would you need to talk to and what would you tell them? And, of course, how would you start to live your new life?

With what you have read, I hope you now can see that the mind can force you to only see the hatred in the world, or make you only see the love. When it happened to me, it was a game-changer, and my mind turned into a very dangerous weapon that went down the some pretty scary roads. But as you know, I eventually made it back onto the right path.

CPSIA information can be obtained
at www.ICGtesting.com
Printed in the USA
BVHW081309031221
623053BV00001B/6